Making Sense of Statistics in Healthcare

Anna Hart

Principal Lecturer in Statistics,
University of Central Lancashire

Radcliffe Medical Press

©2001 Anna Hart
Cartoons ©2001 Dave Colton www.cartoonist.net

Radcliffe Medical Press Ltd
18 Marcham Road, Abingdon, Oxon OX14 1AA

British Library Cataloguing in Publication Data

A catalogue record for this book is available from the British Library.

ISBN 1 85775 472 7

Typeset by Advance Typesetting Ltd, Oxfordshire
Printed and bound by TJ International Ltd, Padstow, Cornwall

Contents

Preface

Not another book about statistics? Yes and no.

This is a book for people who want to be able to make sense of published studies, or to embark on their own studies, without getting bogged down by the details of how to use specific methods. It gives an insight into how statisticians view data and research, and into what they do. It is virtually formula free, and does not describe the mechanics of any techniques, but it is packed with ideas and examples. Surveys have shown that people generally do not understand the basic principles of statistical analysis,[1,2] and I can confirm this from my own experience. There is an argument[3] that it is more important to have a good grasp of 'what' rather than of 'how'. In other words, it is better to have a conceptual understanding of the statistical principles, what to ask and what to look for, rather than a detailed knowledge of a restricted set of specific techniques. Therefore this book discusses statistical concepts in the context of real studies. Most of the data used are real or realistic, although some artificial data are employed to provide extreme examples. I apologise if you think that all of the data should be real. Since the material is designed to be 'friendly', some of the more complicated ideas are identified without giving details or strict accuracy. If you want to know more about specific methods and issues you will need to consult a more technical book, of which there are many available.[4–7] If you like interacting with a computer you may find it useful to explore some of the concepts through experimentation and games. A good example is *Statistics for the Terrified*, which is recommended by the BMA.[8]

A major theme is that you have to combine formal results with common and clinical sense – too many people believe that here is 'a method' to give them the answer. Statistical science is not like that. It is qualitative judgement, not mathematical proof. However, this qualitative aspect makes statistical analyses perplexing to many people. Statisticians must take some of the blame for the way in which they present our subject.[9] I hope that this book is a fair and helpful reflection of statistical science in practice.

Data are everywhere, and we are in danger of being swamped by them. Computers allow gigabytes of numbers to be stored and churned out. There are hundreds of journals, masses of information and disinformation on the Internet, and envelopes of advertising blurb. Clinical governance means that we have to be able to select the best information and make use of it in practice. Evidence-based medicine requires us to access the evidence – evidence from data. However, medical data are notoriously messy. Subjects drop out of studies, fail to attend for appointments, forget to answer questions or complete diaries, or react in unpredictable ways. Moreover, even the best-designed study is likely to have its limitations. Therefore you need to have the confidence to read critically. This book is designed to build that confidence.

In this book the term 'data' refers to numerical data. I am a statistician, so I do quantitative research. That does not mean that I have no time for qualitative research – quite the contrary. It can be very important, especially when finding out about patients' views and priorities. However, I have never done any qualitative research in healthcare, so I cannot write about it. In contrast, I spend a lot of my working time dealing with healthcare data, and I love it. I hope that I can convey some of that enthusiasm to you. Statisticians and statistics have the reputation of being dry, boring and almost dishonest. Yet statistics is a really exciting subject, and quantitative research is truly exciting.

The plan of the book is as follows.

Chapter 1   describes different study designs; this is really important.

Chapter 2   describes different types of data.

Chapter 3   tells you how to interpret charts and graphs and how to detect cheating.

Chapter 4   outlines summary statistics.

Chapter 5   discusses the normal distribution. This is rather technical and can be either skimmed or omitted on a first reading.

Chapter 6   defines the ubiquitous P-value, and shows why confidence intervals are preferable. The latter part can be omitted on a first reading.

Chapter 7   describes the relationships between variables. There are some important ideas here.

Chapter 8   tells you how to read the literature, and defines the common terminology of evidence-based medicine.

Chapter 9   gives advice on how to liaise with a statistician. You can omit this chapter if you do not need to work with statisticians.

The content has been influenced by my personal experience of teaching and consultancy. I have noted the common problems that people encounter with statistics. Many of the examples and ideas are based on real projects in which I have been involved. In addition, the book draws on a number of published papers. You do not need to have access to these papers, but it might help if you could get hold of them. The *British Medical Journal* papers are all available on the World-Wide Web.

When I was new to applied statistics I would have liked a book like this to help demystify what I found very confusing. I hope that it helps you. Please let me know how you get on.

My thanks are due to Dr Chris Sutton and Dr Adrian White for their helpful feedback on the first draft of this book. They greatly improved its quality.

However, the views expressed are mine. Sadly, there will still be errors, for which I take full responsibility and apologise most sincerely.

Finally, I wish you all the very best with your projects.

Anna Hart
March 2001
ahart@uclan.ac.uk

About the author

Anna Hart is the Principal Lecturer in Statistics in the Faculty of Science at the University of Central Lancashire in Preston, and is also an honorary fellow at the University of Exeter. She has a strong interest in practical problems, specifically in medical statistics. Over the years she has had experience of explaining statistical concepts to students and practitioners from a range of backgrounds, many of whom find the subject daunting. One of her favourite creations is an undergraduate module for non-statisticians called *Lying with Numbers?* She acts as a consultant advising on the design and analysis of clinical studies. A variety of happy and less happy experiences in teaching and consultancy have informed this book.

This book is dedicated with much love to Rebekah Shona,
variously known as Gip, Jake or a wide-mouthed frog.
May she learn that I am not crazy all the time!

CHAPTER ONE

Prevention is better than cure

Statistical science is the science of evidence – evidence from data. It is used to evaluate evidence where there is uncertainty or variability in the data. Biological and medical studies are beset with variability. For example, your temperature and blood pressure will vary slightly over time even if you are fit and healthy, two people with the same complaint may respond differently to the same treatment, and a group of people who are exposed to a toxin will not all react in the same way. Statistical science allows you to *describe* what you expect to happen, and also to *quantify the uncertainty* associated with those expectations. Statistics is about the collection and analysis of data. Deciding which data to collect, why and how is a really key issue. Put simply, the *design* of a study is critically important, just as prevention is better than cure. You can analyse the data from a well-designed study, even if they are messy and incomplete, but there may be little you can usefully do with data from an ill-designed study. Since healthcare studies usually involve patients, it is completely unethical to embark on an ill thought out study.

In fact, ethical issues beset studies involving patients. Therefore each study needs a protocol – a detailed description – which serves as a quality control tool for the study. There are several reasons for this. Writing a detailed protocol disciplines one to think carefully about one's research question and the objectives of the study, and hence reduces the likelihood of a poorly thought out design. The document should be unambiguous and hence minimise misunderstandings or false assumptions among members of the research team. It is the means of communicating the detailed ideas to other researchers, and is essential for peer review. During the course of the study the existence of the protocol should discourage conscious or subconscious 'cheating' whereby the researchers deviate from the original plan in order to investigate some other idea that occurs to them, or to implement a different procedure because it seems easier, cheaper or in some way preferable. The protocol will need to be approved by an ethics committee. Approval will almost certainly require the participating patients to give their written informed consent. That means that they are given full details about the study, they have a right to withdraw at any time, and they agree to the terms of the study. A protocol cannot be drawn up without a detailed design.

This chapter describes the basic characteristics of study designs in health-care research. At the end you should be able to:

* distinguish between observational and experimental studies
* describe the main characteristics of a randomised controlled trial
* outline the relative merits of other designs.

Where does it all begin?

You need a reason to collect data. Technically you need a research question and research objectives, but where do these come from? They may come from reading existing publications. The published literature might contain case reports of a few patients. Such case studies or case series often suggest research questions for further investigation. Often the ideas come from ideas or 'hunches' in someone's mind, usually as a result of their having been inquisitive and observant. The observation might be informal (e.g. daily observation of patients). One problem with this can be that even the best scientists can be biased, taking more notice of the evidence which supports their personal beliefs and ignoring that which contradicts them.

More formally the observation might take the form of qualitative research. Typically this consists of an in-depth study of a relatively small number of patients or subjects. The observer starts from a neutral position and lets the 'evidence speak for itself'. Some examples of qualitative methods include observation, interviews and focus groups. These methods collect information about feelings, priorities, problems, reactions and much more.

Suppose, then, that you have such a question in your mind – you are contemplating doing some research. At this stage it is essential to establish what is already known about the subject. After all, you are unlikely to know everything about it. Someone might already have answered your question or a related one. No healthcare research should be undertaken for the amusement of the researcher – it must be for the advancement of useful knowledge. You need to conduct a literature search using an appropriate database such as Medline.[1] You need to obtain and carefully *read* papers of interest. This helps to prevent your repeating mistakes, and it should also tell you whether it is worthwhile pursuing your idea. It might also help you to design your study, or to refine your research question.

The need for designed studies

Once you have a question that is worth asking, you need to think about how you will collect evidence. There is no shortage of anecdotal 'evidence'. For example, people might pontificate about the danger of television programmes that show attempted suicides. No doubt you could find a person who had taken an overdose and who would claim that they had been adversely influenced by such a programme, another person who would claim that they had been deterred from a suicide attempt by the same programme, and a third person who would say that they had not been influenced one way or the other. The three could sit down in a studio and debate the question for as long as you liked, but you could never reach a conclusion about what you could reasonably expect overall from *all* television viewers. Similarly, most people know someone who was a heavy smoker for years and yet lived to a ripe old age and did not die of cancer or cardiovascular problems. This single example would not mean that smoking is safe. There are many people who swear by a potion or apparently odd treatment for an ailment. The testimony from one person does not justify recommending the 'wonder-cure' for all and sundry.

If the evidence is to be useful it has to be collected in a systematic way – you decide *what you want to collect* and *how best to obtain it*. You need a plan. One of the major problems with the above examples is that the people may not be *representative*. When you conduct a study you usually want the results to be generalisable, even though you will only study some people. The *population* is the whole set of people (or items) about which you want information. This is usually far too large to study. The *sample* is the group of people (or items) that you actually study, and you can study the sample in some detail. It is fairly obvious that if the sample is *representative* (i.e. typical) of the population then there is a good chance that any results you obtain from the sample will be valid for the population. However, if the sample is not typical of the population, the results really only tell you about that sample. There is no way that you can correct the results for information which you do not have. Thus the choice of a study sample is critical for the quality of the study.

Randomised controlled trial

Observation is the process of watching what is happening without interfering with it. In contrast, *experiments* are the basis of many scientific enquiries. In an experiment you *do something* (e.g. give a piece of advice or administer a treatment) and then *measure what happens*. Suppose, for example, that you have the following research question:

Does drug X arrest the progression of motor neurone disease (MND)?

We shall assume that there is some good reason to suspect that drug X might be effective, but insufficient evidence to justify advocating its general use. How do you set about designing a suitable study? You would need to decide on the recommended dose of the drug. You would also need to decide on a method for measuring the progression of MND. This might be an overall measure of muscle strength or disability. In statistical terminology this would be an example of a *variable*. A variable is simply some characteristic, subject to variability, which is being measured. For this particular study the chosen variable would have to be one that any expert would accept as a valid measure of the severity of the disease, and capable of detecting change. Then you would need to select your sample of patients. It needs to be established that they do indeed have MND, and you might want to eliminate patients with other diseases or complications or those at high risk of side-effects. Next you would need to decide on the number of patients to study and the period of time involved. You would consult the literature to help you with all such decisions. In practice, you would need to obtain approval from an ethics committee, as well as written informed consent from the patients, but let us assume that this would be forthcoming.

Such a study conducted on one group of patients would in fact be of little value (and should not gain ethics committee approval). The reason is that you would have nothing with which to compare the results of this group. How would you know what to expect from this group of patients over this period of time at this stage in their disease if they had *not* been taking the drug? You cannot know. Thus if overall they all seemed to deteriorate, you could not conclude that the drug had been ineffective, because their deterioration might have been worse without the drug. Conversely, if they did not deteriorate overall, you could not attribute this to the drug. The patients will know that they are in a study, and that they are being monitored. As a result they might take better care of themselves, or have a more positive psychological outlook. It is possible, even if you think it unlikely, that the apparent effect could be the result of their being in the study rather than it being a specific effect of the drug.

Such an experiment requires a *control group* – that is, a group for comparison. In fact, early on in the design of the study you should ask the question:

> I am interested in the effectiveness of drug X. Effectiveness in comparison with what?

With the exception of the active drug component, you want the control group to have exactly the same experience as the treatment group. This is because any difference in outcomes between the two groups can be attributed to *any* aspect or aspects differing between the two groups. For example, if all of the control group were males and all of the treatment group were females, you would not be able to distinguish between a possible effect of gender and that of the drug. Therefore the control group must take some form of treatment or pseudotreatment. If there is no accepted drug for MND, then you can use a *placebo*. A placebo is a substance that is indistinguishable from the active drug, but which is actually inert. If there is a recognised drug then it would be unethical to withhold it, and you might give one group the recognised drug and the other group the new drug. Alternatively, you might give both groups the recognised drug and in addition give one group the new drug and the other group the placebo. This is called a *combination therapy*. Note that these two scenarios would be addressing different research questions about the new drug X. One study is asking questions about its effectiveness when taken in conjunction with the recognised drug, and the other is asking about its effectiveness when taken on its own. The issue of which design was the more appropriate one would depend on your objectives and background knowledge about drug X. In general, the research question you ask is related to the choice of control group as well as to the choice of treatment and treatment group.

Let us assume that it is acceptable to give a placebo to the control group and drug X to the treatment group. There is now another question that needs to be answered. How are the patients to be allocated to the two groups? You cannot ask for volunteers. If you did so, you would end up with the people who preferred to take the active drug in one group and those who preferred not to take it in the other. This would defeat the object of having the placebo, because it would introduce a difference between the two groups. For example, if you let a clinician or nurse decide, then you might obtain an imbalance between the two groups. A clinician who was sympathetic to the needs of the patients might be inclined to put the more disabled patients in the active drug group, and this could mask any benefits of the drug. The only fair way to allocate individuals to the groups is by using the principle of chance.

You do the equivalent of tossing a coin. In practice, you do not use an informal procedure such as tossing a coin or drawing names out of a hat. You must have a system that is open to audit – that is, capable of being checked afterwards. You use random number tables or a computer to achieve such a system. Assuming that you want groups of approximately equal sizes, there would be a probability of $\frac{1}{2}$ that any particular person is allocated to the treatment group. Then there will be no systematic differences between the two groups. This process is called *randomisation* (an example is given in Appendix A).

Thus the patients would know that they were in a study and that they were taking either drug X or a placebo, but they would not know which substance they were taking. A further aspect of the ideal design is that all study participants – the subjects, carers, assessors (the people measuring the deterioration) and those managing the data – should also be unaware of which group the patient has been allocated to. This avoids their being prejudiced by their view of the potential benefit of drug X. Such a design is described as *double-blind*.

We can briefly summarise as follows.

- *Controlled* means that there is a control group.
- *Randomised* means that patients are allocated to treatment or control groups by chance.
- *Double-blind* means that neither the patient nor the clinical staff knows which group a patient has been allocated to.

This type of study is called a double-blind randomised controlled trial. A randomised controlled trial is often abbreviated to RCT.

This type of study is a true experiment. The experimenter controls the *factor* of interest, namely the drug. (A factor is a variable that can take a few distinct values.) The double-blind RCT is one of the best possible designs. In therapeutics it is the *only sure way to show that a therapy causes the observed effect*. As will be discussed later, other designs are open to alternative interpretations. Although it is 'ideal', it is not always feasible. For example, double-blinding may not be possible or even desirable. If you are comparing two different casts for torn ligaments in the ankle, the patients cannot be literally blinded in order to prevent them knowing which type of cast they have. Similarly, double-blinding is impossible for surgical procedures or behavioural studies.

In practice, usage of the terminology for blinding is somewhat inconsistent. Some people describe studies as double-blind if neither the patients nor the assessors know the treatment allocation, but the carers do. The term *single-blinding* is commonly used to describe a study in which the patient does not know which group they are in, whereas the assessor does, but some people use the term to describe the opposite scenario. Common sense needs to be applied, the aim being to have as much blinding as possible in order to reduce the influence of prior beliefs on findings – that is, psychological effects. Blinding is therefore very important if the variables being measured are subjective (e.g. level of pain). Furthermore, the assessor should be blinded wherever possible.

Some researchers regard this approach as naive, because psychological effects can be an important component of overall treatment effects. Furthermore, the size of specific treatment effects might *depend* on non-specific factors such as the therapist, the clinical setting, the patient's beliefs or the information given. A study that minimised the placebo effects might therefore bear little resemblance to clinical practice, where the effects of placebos may well be maximised.[2] Such researchers would conduct pragmatic trials. None the less, most RCTs employ blinding.

Simple randomisation is not always used. Sometimes extra efforts are made to ensure that the two groups are as similar or *balanced* as possible with regard to a number of important variables. Randomisation will not ensure that the two groups are balanced, but merely that it is impossible to know what the imbalance will be. For example, there may be a higher proportion of males in one group. Some people prefer modifications to simple randomisation that attempt to ensure balance.[3–5] You try to balance groups with respect to variables that you believe to be influential on the outcome of interest. However, balancing is not very important for large studies, and many researchers risk designing overly complicated studies by attempting to balance with respect to too many variables.[5] There are several variations on the basic design of an RCT. Standard texts[4,6–8] give practical details and advice, and the basic principles are as outlined here.

Avoiding bias

The principles outlined in the previous section are all designed to reduce *bias*. Bias is systematic (as opposed to random) error. There are several sources of bias in a study:[9]

- *selection bias* occurs when there are differences between the two treatment groups irrespective of and before any treatment effects
- *performance bias* occurs when the two groups receive different care in addition to the treatment difference under study
- *attrition bias* occurs when there are different patterns of dropout from the study in the two groups
- *detection bias* occurs when there are systematic differences in the assessments of the two groups.

Blinding is the principal strategy used to minimise the last three of these biases. Selection bias is minimised to a certain extent by randomisation, but also by *allocation concealment*. This means that the allocation system should be designed in such a way that the person who is recruiting subjects to the study does not know in advance to which treatment group the next subject will be assigned. They should make a decision about the eligibility of the subject before the allocation is made, and then they should not be able to change either the allocation or the decision about eligibility. As a general rule, the person who generated the allocation scheme should not administer it. A common way of achieving this is to have a series of consecutively numbered, sealed, opaque envelopes, each of which contains a treatment allocation. Other details are given in the *Cochrane Handbook*,[9] which states that 'preventing foreknowledge of treatment assignment is crucially important', and that 'one of the most important factors that may lead to bias and distort treatment comparisons is that which can result from the way that comparison groups are assembled'.

Prospective cohort study

You cannot force people to take part in an RCT, because it may do them harm. If they agree to take part they have the right to withdraw at any time. For some research questions it is impossible or unethical to conduct an RCT at all. For example, if you are interested in the effect on health of a toxin or risk factor, you cannot even invite people to be exposed to it. The classical example is smoking – you cannot ask people to smoke. Since the risk factor is not under the control of the researcher, such a study will be observational, not experimental. The best type of observational study is *prospective*. In a prospective study a group or groups of people are chosen and followed forward in time. Such a group is called a *cohort*. Typically, you first measure the subjects' exposure to the risk factor and then follow them, monitoring for development of the disease. Prospective studies can be costly if there is likely to be a long time interval between exposure to the risk factor and development of the disease or outcome. Moreover, if the incidence of the disease is low, you might need to study very large samples of people in order to observe sufficient cases of the disease.

Even if you overcome these problems, and you find that the likelihood of developing the disease is greater in the exposed group, you cannot conclude that the risk factor *causes* the disease. All you can show is an *association* between the two. This is because you have no control over exposure to the risk factor. It can always be argued, however implausible you may consider it, that there is another variable that causes people to be exposed to the risk factor and which also causes the disease. For years this was argued about smoking and cancer. Maybe, it was said, there were genetic effects which made people more prone to smoke, and which also made them more susceptible to cancer. Similar arguments could be used for any risk factor. If living near electricity cables or nuclear installations is associated with an illness, perhaps certain types of people tend to live in those types of locations and also tend to get the illness. Observational studies cannot establish cause and effect. However, they are useful, and prospective cohort studies can be used to estimate the probabilities of contracting the disease with or without the risk factor, perhaps taking into account other variables. Chapter 8 describes the characteristics of observational studies where evidence for causality is strong.

Case–control study

The prospective cohort study selects subjects on the basis of their exposure to a risk factor and follows them forward. If this is impractical, then a *retrospective* study could be considered. In a retrospective study groups are chosen and followed *back* in time. Usually the groups are chosen not on the basis of exposure to the risk factor but on the basis of disease. You choose two groups of people – the *cases* have the disease of interest and the *controls* do not. Looking back you see how many individuals in each group had been exposed to the risk factor. However, you are likely to have a disproportionate number of cases in your sample relative to the population, so this method cannot usually be used to estimate the probabilities of contracting the disease with or without exposure to the risk factor. It *can* be used to determine whether the likelihood of contracting the disease is the same with or without the risk factor. Furthermore, in many case–control studies it is possible to make statements such as 'You are three times more likely to contract X if you have been exposed to Y'.

As with cohort studies, it is impossible to establish cause and effect. Moreover, there are other practical problems with these studies, some of which are listed below.

- Selection of controls is difficult. They need to be free of the disease, but they and the cases need to have had similar exposure to the risk factor under investigation and to any other known risk factors.
- There may be differences between cases and controls that are related to the disease but not to the risk factor.
- The passage of time might mean that it is difficult to establish exposure – people might have different abilities or levels of recall in the groups.
- Cases might be more likely to admit to exposure than controls.
- Assessors may not be blinded to disease status, and this might influence the way in which they interview the subjects.

The design of a case–control study requires great care. More details of case–control and cohort studies are given in classic texts.[10–13] The elimination of bias in such studies is also important.[9]

Cross-sectional studies – surveys

In a prospective study (sometimes called a *longitudinal* study) subjects are followed over time. In contrast, *cross-sectional* studies measure outcomes at a single point in time for a number of individuals. They tend to be less informative, as it is impossible to distinguish between variability in the data due to changes over time and that due to differences between individuals.

One common type of cross-sectional study is a *survey* (although some surveys are implemented as part of a longitudinal study). Surveys are often administered by a questionnaire, and are very popular with many researchers. However, a critical problem is non-response. You might exercise all the care in the world when choosing the sample of individuals to whom you give the questionnaire, but if only certain types of people respond you will not have replies that are typical of the population. Typically, response rates are poor for postal surveys administered to healthy people. Response rates of 40% are considered to be quite good in some areas, and they can be as low as 15% or 20%. These could be responses from individuals who feel very strongly about the topic of research, and then the results will be biased towards those people. If you intend to conduct a survey, you must think very carefully about how you are going to ensure a high response rate. The best journals refuse to publish the results of surveys with low response rates.

For surveys, the *sampling frame* is the list of the whole population of interest, and it can be difficult to obtain this. The sample is drawn from this list. One method is to take a simple *random sample* chosen by random numbers. Basically you decide on the proportion of the population that you wish to survey and then select them using random numbers. A simple example is given in Appendix B. Other sampling methods are used to meet special requirements.

The questions in the questionnaire must be clear, unambiguous and understandable. The person answering the question must have the same understanding of what it is asking as the person who wrote it. This means that unless you are using a questionnaire whose validity is already established for the actual use you have in mind, you must *pilot* it – that is, you need to give it to a smaller but typical set of respondents and obtain their feedback. You may need to modify the questionnaire before carrying out your full survey. The many practical problems associated with questionnaires are described in specialist texts.[14–16]

If you send the questionnaire to the whole population, then you are conducting a *census*. Although the analysis will be slightly different, the pitfalls are similar, and you still need to ensure a high response rate.

Reliability studies

Another type of study is becoming increasingly important in healthcare, namely the reliability study. For example, you might have developed a method for rating, say, 'willingness to change' in obese patients who want to lose weight. This method is a 'tool' that can be used by several 'assessors'. You might be interested in the following aspects related to reliability:

- the agreement of results using the same assessor at two different times
- the agreement of results using different assessors at the same time
- the agreement between this tool and another established one.

The designs of studies such as this can get quite complicated, but they all employ the basic principles of experimental design. As with any study, you must ensure that your samples are representative of the populations of interest. Here this involves thinking about the choice of subjects to be assessed, the choice of assessors, the choice of methods used and also the clinical setting in which the assessments are to take place. You must make sure that the design allows the aspect of interest to be observed and measured, and that it is not confused with some other effect. You must also be clear about how you expect your results to be generalised. For example, are you interested in the reliability of the specific assessors in your study or of assessors in general? It is important to minimise contamination effects (e.g. assessors knowing the results of one method while using the other, or the subject responding differently to later assessments because of learning effects).

Some experimental designs appear superficially to be the same, but might in fact measure different effects and require different analyses. You really need advice from someone who knows about experimental design and how best to juggle the many factors in the study.

Examples

Below are some examples of studies that illustrate the various different designs. The results of some of these studies will be discussed later in the book.

Case study A

Randomised controlled trials are not just used for the study of drugs. A group of researchers in Wiltshire, UK, used an RCT design to evaluate the safety and effectiveness of a nurse telephone consultation system in out-of-hours primary care.[17] The 'treatment' was the nurse consultation system augmenting standard service, using trained nurses backed up by a decision support system. The 'control' was the standard service. The aim was to determine whether there was an equivalent number of adverse events (e.g. deaths within 7 days of contact, emergency hospital admission within 24 hours) for each system. The study ran over a period of 1 year, in order to avoid bias from seasonal effects. The year was divided into 2-weekly intervals. Within each interval of 2 weeks the 'treatment' was allocated at random so that one Tuesday night had the nurse consultation system and the other had the standard service, one Thursday night had the nurse consultation system and the other had the standard service, and so on. The general practitioners did not know in advance which system was in place for any session, nor did the patients phoning in. Without knowing the details of the design it would have been very difficult to predict at any time which system was in place. Note how the researchers tried to make the results generalisable. They ran the study for a whole year and ensured a balance between the allocation of different systems to the time slots. They also applied randomisation in the allocation of systems to time slots, and tried to ensure as much blinding as possible.

Case study B

A prospective cohort study was undertaken in Avon, UK.[18] The researchers were looking at the association between postnatal catch-up growth and obesity in childhood. Some infants who are small or thin at birth exhibit 'catch-up' growth in the first 2 years of life. The researchers selected a sample of infants and measured them at birth, every 4 months to 12 months, every 6 months to 4 years, and at 5 years. They had complete data for 848 infants, and looked at associations between catch-up growth and obesity. This could not have been investigated by an experiment, as birth weight could not be controlled. A longitudinal study is quite appropriate here.

Case study C

Researchers in Norway used a prospective cohort study to study mental health problems in junior house-officers.[19] They used a postal questionnaire survey which was sent to medical students in their graduating semester and then again after 1 year when they were junior house-doctors. They sent questionnaires to students at all four medical schools in Norway, and obtained a response rate of 83% for the first survey and 58% for the second one (i.e. 71% of those who responded the first time). They were able to perform cross-sectional analyses – for example, to look at the prevalence of mental health problems and to examine possible relationships between working conditions and mental health problems. They were also able to conduct a longitudinal analysis looking at associations between factors in the final year of medical school and subsequent development of mental health problems.

Case study D

A special type of longitudinal study called an *interrupted time series* was employed in a different study.[20] The objective was to determine whether the depiction of a serious overdose in a television drama altered the nature of presentations of self-poisoning at hospitals in the UK. This is another case where an experiment was not feasible, but a prospective longitudinal study was. The study involved 49 Accident and Emergency departments and psychiatric services in the UK. Each participating centre monitored the presentations of patients in the 3 weeks before the broadcast and also in the 3 weeks after it. This was possible because advance notice was given of the broadcast. The weeks before the broadcast were like a 'control' group, and those after the broadcast were like the 'treatment' group. The study compared the 'before' and 'after' data to look for possible effects of the programme.

Case study E

A case–control study was used by researchers in the USA[21] who were investigating the association between exposure to sunlight and death from multiple sclerosis. Data were obtained from death certificates between 1984 and 1995 in 24 states. The cases were deaths from multiple sclerosis, and the controls were deaths from other causes, excluding cancer and some other neurological disorders (for comparative purposes they also studied the association between exposure to sunlight and non-melanoma skin cancer). An attempt was made to match the cases and controls with regard to age, and the analysis took into account other influences such as gender, race and socioeconomic status. Exposure to sunlight was determined by the state of residence recorded on the death certificate, and subjects were only included if they resided in the same solar radiation region at birth and death. The authors were aware of the limitations of case–control studies, and describe their study as 'exploratory'. Specifically, they note the possibility that the patterns of exposure to sunlight might have been different between cases and controls.

Case study F

An example of a cross-sectional study is provided by researchers investigating an association between eating disorders and type I diabetes in adolescent girls.[22] Girls aged 12–19 years who had had type I diabetes for at least a year were identified from clinics in three Canadian cities. A comparison group, matched for age, was identified from schools. There were approximately three times as many controls as diabetics. Each girl completed a self-report package, including previously validated tools for identifying eating disorders, and their body mass indices were calculated. This information was used to identify those who might have eating disorders, and they were asked to attend a semi-structured diagnostic interview. This interview method had already been validated. The interviewers could not be blinded to diabetic status, but they were blinded to status for eating disorders. This was achieved by also inviting a set of girls who appeared to have no symptoms of eating disorders to be interviewed. Participation rates were high, with 84% of diabetic girls agreeing to participate and 74% of the eligible controls, although not all of these were selected. This study gives a 'snapshot' picture of the association between diabetes and eating disorders.

Case study G

A group of dentists conducted a different type of study.[23] They were interested in dentists' agreement on the treatment of asymptomatic impacted third molar teeth. They used specially prepared case-notes for 23 patients. A random sample of 90 dentists was taken from the 391 dentists listed in two district health authorities in north-west England. An appointment was made and the dentist viewed the notes and made a recommendation. This was repeated a month later, but at the first assessment the dentist was unaware that the second assessment would take place. This was in order to avoid carry-over problems due to memorising responses. A total of 74 dentists took part. This design allowed two types of agreement to be measured. First, it was possible to measure the *agreement between* dentists. This was done twice – at each of the assessments – giving two measures of agreement. Secondly, it was possible to measure the *reliability* of each dentist's decisions over time, giving 74 different measures – one for each dentist. This was a fairly simple design, but it illustrates a study of two types of reliability.

Case study H

Similar techniques were used to validate a questionnaire.[24] The study was a cross-sectional survey in Edinburgh. A sample was drawn from the computerised age–sex registers of 12 general practices in the city, which covered a range of geographical and socio-economic areas. The objective was to establish the relationships between age, gender, symptoms in the lower limbs and the presence of varicose veins. Details of symptoms were elicited by means of a self-administered questionnaire. Before using it the researchers needed to know how reliable the questionnaire was, so they circulated it on two occasions, 6 weeks apart, to 62 individuals in their university department. This enabled them to measure the level of agreement between answers from the same people but at different times. The period of 6 weeks was chosen in order to eliminate memory effects, but to ensure that symptoms would be as identical as possible at the two times.

This study had another interesting feature. The researchers did not take a simple random sample from the registers. They invited equal numbers of men and women to take part. Moreover, they did not take a simple random sample, but rather they sampled within age bands (e.g. 25–34 years, 35–44 years). This was because they wanted to compare the effects of gender and age. A simple random sample might have resulted in a very small proportion of certain age groups. The method used here is called *stratified* sampling, with random samples being taken from subsets of the sampling frame rather than one sample being taken from the entire sampling frame. This method is commonly used to compare subgroups of a population.

Case studies A to F will be referred to again in the following chapters.

Summary

Design is a critical stage of any study. It can be very time-consuming, but is essential. You should include expert help at a very early stage. The main points covered in this chapter are as follows.

- A designed experiment, typically an RCT, is the best design for establishing cause and effect.
- Blinding is used to minimise or eliminate bias.
- Observational studies cannot establish cause and effect.
- A prospective study follows subjects forward in time, but can be costly.
- A retrospective study follows subjects back in time, but is difficult to design.
- Surveys require careful questionnaire design, and low response rates are a problem.
- Reliability studies require application of the principles of experimental design.

CHAPTER TWO

A multitude
of types

Data are the building blocks of statistics. If you have no data then you can have no statistics! When collecting data, people use instruments or machines to make objective measurements, they collect facts and figures about events, and they ask patients about their opinions and feelings. There is therefore a multitude of different *types* of data. If you do not understand the nature of your data, you are in danger of analysing them incorrectly. After all, the computer or calculator has no idea about data, so it is critical that the person pressing the buttons is able to judge the sense of what they are doing. This chapter explores some of the different types of data that you are likely to encounter. The material is largely motivated by the study of mental health problems among young doctors[1] described in Case Study C.

At the end of this chapter you should be able to:

* recognise different types of data
* identify some of the ways in which different types of data can be handled.

Background study

Four researchers in Norway were aware that previous studies had identified an increased prevalence of mental health problems among physicians, especially in their early postgraduate years. They set out to investigate the factors that influence the mental health of junior house-officers in Norway. To this end they decided to survey all medical students graduating in 1993 and 1994 in Norway. All such students received a postal questionnaire during their last term and another one a year later, after their first postgraduate year in hospital. This is an example of a *prospective cohort study*.

Their questionnaire contained many questions, which elicited different types of data. The published paper contains several tables summarising the answers to the questions and the relationships between them.

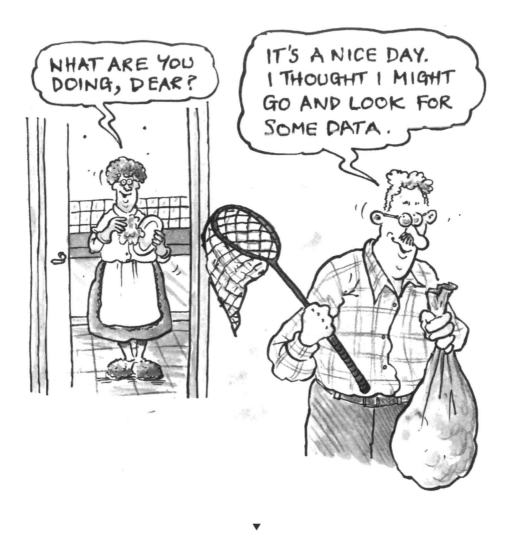

Binary data

A question fundamental to the study was 'Have you had mental health problems during internship?'

The possible answers were 'yes' and 'no'. This is an example of a *binary* (sometimes referred to as *dichotomous*) response. All this means is that there are two possible answers, which can be coded as 0 and 1 (just as binary numbers are stored in computers). The answers could just as well be coded as N and Y, or as 1 and 2. You need two different symbols to describe the answers, and the symbols may actually be meaningless in themselves.

Ordinal data

If the answer to the question about mental health problems was 'yes', then the doctor was asked to answer the following question: 'Have you sought/received help for this?'

The doctor had five possible answers from which to choose one response:

1 had mental health problems of no importance
2 have not sought help, although I have been in need of this
3 have consulted GP
4 have consulted psychologist/psychiatrist
5 have been admitted to mental hospital.

These answers indicate increasing severity of the acknowledged mental health problem. Having been admitted to hospital reflects a worse condition than having merely consulted a psychologist or psychiatrist, and this in turn is worse than having consulted a general practitioner. In other words, there is a natural order to the answers. Such data are described as *ordinal*. The numbers 1 to 5 are a fairly natural way of labelling or coding the replies. Reply 4 is more serious than reply 2, in the same way that the number 4 is greater than the number 2. However, the same relationship could be reflected by different coding systems. For example, the codes could just as easily be 100, 200, 300, 400 and 500, or even 610, 620, 630, 640 and 650. It would *not* be sensible to code them as 100, 50, 20, 75 and 200. However, it is important to recognise that the numbers are labels, and not necessarily a *direct* measure of severity. For example, a problem described by the answer 4 is not necessarily twice as severe as one described by the answer 2. Moreover, it is not obvious that the difference between answers 1 and 2 reflects the same type of difference as that between answers 3 and 4. The answers have the same *order* as the numbers, but they may not share the other properties of those numbers.

Another binary variable

The doctors were asked about their marital status, and the possible answers were as follows:

1 unmarried
2 cohabiting
3 married
4 separated
5 divorced.

Here again there are five options, but the situation is somewhat different. First, the answers are not *mutually exclusive*. For example, a doctor could be both divorced and a cohabitant. Such a person would tick more than one answer. Furthermore, the answers do not have a natural ranking. Therefore the question really consists of several separate questions, each of which has a binary response. However, the answers are not *independent* of each other. For example, a doctor who is married cannot also be unmarried. In fact, the researchers collapsed the answers into one binary variable by coding the replies from all of the doctors who were either married or cohabiting as 1 and the remainder as 0. This discriminated between those who lived with a partner and those who did not. In general, the earlier you decide how you are going to code the data the better. If you do not think carefully about this you may end up collecting the wrong type of answers. Of course, all this requires you to think carefully about *why* you are collecting the data in the first place. What do you hope to do with it? What is your research question?

Continuous variables

The paper states that 'age was measured as a continuous variable'. A *continuous* variable is one which can take decimal values, and whose accuracy is only limited by how it is measured. You often use an instrument (e.g. weighing scales) to measure a continuous variable. Typical examples are height and weight. These are sometimes recorded to the nearest unit of measurement (e.g. cm or g). Age is clearly a continuous variable. However, few people would describe their age as 28.12 years – they would say 28 years. In general, adults state their age in years only (children are often far more enthusiastic about giving you the extra fraction of a year). This is potentially misleading if the actual age is 28 years 364 days. Although colloquially one would describe this as 28 years, mathematically it would be more accurate to round it up to 29 years. In order to record an age accurately, you normally ask for an age in years and months, or for the current date and date of birth so that you can work out the exact age yourself. Again, the accuracy that you require will depend on the intended use of the data. In this paper, the researchers do not provide the details of how they obtained age as a continuous variable.

Numbers are the only sensible way of recording continuous variables. Moreover, the numbers usually obey the rules of arithmetic. A weight of 12 kg is twice as heavy as one of 6 kg, and the actual (not percentage) difference between 10 kg and 11 kg is the same as that between 34 kg and 35 kg. Most continuous variables share these properties. A notable exception is temperature expressed in degrees Centigrade (or Fahrenheit). The temperature 38 degrees Centigrade is not twice as hot as 19 degrees Centigrade (this is because zero degrees is not an absolute zero on this scale). However, care must be exercised. Often continuous variables are recorded to the nearest whole number, and so appear to be *discrete*. It is sometimes very important to distinguish between values like this and those which are by their nature whole numbers.

Discrete variables

For example, in the survey, the Norwegian doctors were asked about their exposure to life events during the previous 12 months. They had a list of 13 events, each of which could induce stress, and which might have been experienced. One such event was the death of a family member or close friend. The researchers state that 'all items were coded 0 or 1 and the variable comprised the sumscore of all variables'. This variable is a count, and could take only the whole numbers 0 to 13. The numbers of items or counts are discrete variables. Other examples could include the number of deaths per year, or the number of patients attending a particular clinic.

Eliciting more complicated data

Another variable that was measured was defined as 'climate for learning in the hospital posts'. The aim was to 'reflect the working atmosphere, especially the need for good learning conditions, of junior house-officers'. The question-naire included ten statements such as:

* my senior is easily available when I am on call
* I am often praised when my work is well done.

For each of these ten statements the doctors were asked to rate how much they agreed with them, as follows:

1   completely untrue
2   mostly untrue
3   partly true
4   mostly true
5   completely true.

This is another example of a 5-point ordinal scale. However, the scores from each statement were added together to give a total score which would be a whole number between 10 and 50. High total scores were deemed to reflect a 'positive perceived climate for learning among the subjects'. This type of approach is common for psychologically related or quality-of-life measures. However, the construction of a suitable instrument like this is by no means straightforward.[2] It needs to be *validated* – that is, it is necessary to show that it does indeed measure what it is intended to measure. Do higher scores really reflect better situations? Is the score capable of measuring change? Does it cover all of the issues known to be relevant? How does it compare with other scoring systems that measure the same characteristic? Is it intended to reflect a patient's or a doctor's assessment of a situation? Would different people measuring the same thing obtain the same value? Would the same person using it on two occasions obtain the same value? As you might imagine, this takes a great deal of time and effort. Nowadays there are many scales available to measure health, disability, quality of life, pain, etc.[3-6] In practice, it is much better to use an existing validated measure than to try to invent one yourself. Care must also be taken if you amend an existing method, as the original validation may no longer hold. This also applies to translations into other languages or uses in different cultures and contexts. A method is validated for a specific purpose – it does not follow that it is valid for a slightly different purpose.

You may wonder whether such a derived score is ordinal or discrete. This is a good question, and the answer depends on the particular score. The characteristics of a score should have been established during its validation. In practice, the scores are often treated as if they were continuous variables.

Scaling responses

The basic scales used in this part of the questionnaire were 5-point scales. Ordinal responses can be elicited on 3-point, 4-point or up to 7-, 8- or 9-point scales. Too many levels will be confusing and irritating for the subject to use, and will only give a semblance of accuracy. On the other hand, a scale which does not allow the subject to discriminate will lead to a loss of information. Five to seven categories are generally considered to be optimal, but in practice it is always a good idea to pilot a question on a few typical subjects to ensure that they can use it.

The term *Likert scale* is very commonly used. Figure 2.1 shows an example of a 7-point Likert-type scale. The subjects are asked to indicate their opinion by rating their *agreement* with a series of statements. The principal feature of such a scale is that the answers are on an agree–disagree continuum. Some

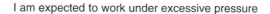

I am expected to work under excessive pressure

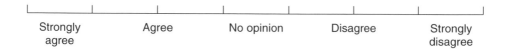

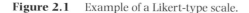
Strongly   Agree   No opinion   Disagree   Strongly
agree   disagree

Figure 2.1   Example of a Likert-type scale.

people argue that the number of tick marks or divisions must match the number of labels, but this rule is not always adhered to. Clearly the example shown in Figure 2.1 does not obey this rule. The scale should, of course, be understandable to the people who are using it.

Another technique that is very popular is a *visual analogue scale* (VAS), an example of which is shown in Figure 2.2.

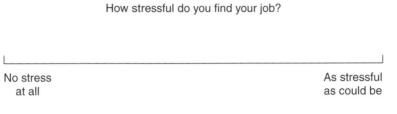

Figure 2.2   Example of a visual analogue scale (VAS).

A VAS consists of a line of fixed length – usually 10 cm – with extreme labels at the ends. Subjects are asked to place a mark such as a cross on the scale to correspond with their opinion or condition. The distance of the cross along the line can be measured as a value, and is therefore a real number. This looks deceptively simple. Does this mean that the variable being measured has similar properties to the continuous variables such as height and weight? The answer is almost certainly no. A scale such as this is usually used to measure subjective opinion or feeling. The repeated answers from an individual may be ordinal, but people may vary in their use of the scale, so the data *between* subjects may not be ordinal at all. Moreover, it is unlikely that a subject will use the scale in a linear manner. People may be very reluctant to mark at the extremes and, as with other ordinal scales, a mark at 4 cm may not indicate a value which is twice that at 2 cm, and it may take more to move a subject from 8 cm to 9 cm than from 5 cm to 6 cm. Although the instrument looks easy to use, some subjects find it quite difficult. Yet again there is a strong case for piloting. Apparent accuracy of the value elicited is of little benefit if you do not know what the numbers mean.

As an illustration, consider the following response of a man who was admitted to a hospital Accident and Emergency department with intense chest pain. The man was asked the following question: 'On a scale of 0 to 10, where 0 is no pain at all and 10 is the worst pain imaginable, how bad is the pain now?' The man replied 'Seven', and then added under his breath, 'It was 110 before'.

Nominal variables

If the Norwegian researchers had asked about the medical school from which the doctors had graduated, they would have collected another type of data. There were four medical schools in Norway. Unless they had some special reason for ordering these four, this variable would have been an example of a *nominal* variable. This is a variable which can take one of several values, but where there is no ranking to those values. They might eventually be coded as numbers in a computer, but the choice of numbers is entirely arbitrary. Other examples of nominal data include ethnic origin, religion and blood type. The coding of nominal data might appear very similar to that of ordinal or discrete data. However, what you can sensibly *do* with the numbers will depend on the type of data.

Recoding

The practice of recoding values into a new binary variable or an ordinal variable with few values (as with marital status in this study) is quite popular. You could measure weight in kg and then recode it as high, medium or low, or you could measure a change in VAS pain score following an operation and code the change as satisfactory or unsatisfactory. Although the resulting data would appear simpler, the simplicity is achieved at the expense of a loss of information. As a general principle, you should retain as much of the information as possible. The analysis of continuous data is in many ways much easier than the analysis of ordinal or binary data. The recoding can be useful for summary statistics, and for meaningful interpretation of results (*see* Chapter 4), but the original data should always be retained. Other methods of recoding include the calculation of ratios and percentages. A primary objective is to collect quality data. For example, suppose that you are interested in collecting data about percentage changes, but that it is easier for subjects to provide 'before' and 'after' values. You should ask them for the data that they could provide accurately and with relative ease, and do the recoding yourself.

Does it matter?

Clearly there are many types of variables. Although it is useful to know how statisticians classify them, it is much more important to understand what a particular variable is, how and why it is measured, and how it can be used. It is vital that you do this in your own research, and equally important that you read research reports and papers critically in order to ascertain whether other people have asked the right questions about their data and variables. Failure to do this may mean that the data collected are not what you think they are, that you fail to record information, that the analysis is nonsense, or that you are unable to answer your initial research question.

Summary

- There are many types of data, and different types can be handled in different ways.
- Binary variables can only have two values (e.g. yes/no, male/female, alive/dead).
- Nominal variables can take several values, and there is no obvious ordering to the values (e.g. hair colour, marital status, blood group).
- Ordinal variables are like nominal variables, but there is a natural ranking to the values (e.g. stage of cancer, degree of pain, level of stress, socio-economic class).
- Discrete variables take numerical values, but their values are restricted. They usually describe counts (e.g. number of children, number of adverse events experienced).
- Continuous variables are measured, and the degree of accuracy is only limited by the measuring instrument (e.g. height, weight, blood pressure).
- Different instruments can be used to measure variables. The instrument must be *valid* and *reliable*. It is best to use an existing validated method, and in any case it is good practice to pilot a method.
- If you do not think carefully about what you are trying to measure and why, you are likely to miss vital information.
- You should check carefully that other people have used a valid and reliable method to elicit what they wished to measure, and that sufficient information is provided about what they measured, how and why.

CHAPTER THREE

A picture speaks a thousand words, or a good few lies!

One message of Chapter 2 was that data should be recorded as measured, and not regrouped without good reason. However, raw data generally consist of an indigestible amount of information. Research questions are answered by summarising the data into numbers or pictures. This necessarily involves a loss of information. The key is to extract the salient features of the data that are relevant to the question being asked. These features then need to be communicated in an unambiguous and meaningful manner. Most people are more comfortable interpreting pictures than tables of figures, and they quickly gain an impression of the main features of a picture. Unfortunately, this fact can be manipulated by the careless or unscrupulous, and charts can give a false impression of the real data. This chapter therefore describes some of the basic charts, and shows you how to avoid being deceived by unfair use of charts.

At the end of this chapter you should be able to

- interpret simple charts and graphs
- examine charts critically and assess their fairness.

Have a go yourself

A good way to investigate the fairness of charts is to try to interpret some of them. Several examples are given below. You should spend a reasonable amount of time looking at each chart, but not substantially more than you would expect to spend looking at them in practice.

Figures 3.1 to 3.4 show four different charts, each of which is accompanied by a short background description and a question. Use the chart to answer the question, and keep a note of your confidence in your answers.

Study 1

A survey of in-patients is regularly conducted at a hospital in order to assess patient satisfaction with the catering service. One of the questions is as follows.

What is your opinion of the temperature of the cooked food?

1   too cold
2   about right
3   too hot.

Figure 3.1 depicts a summary of the answers to this question from the most recent survey.

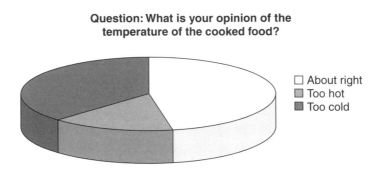

Question: What is your opinion of the temperature of the cooked food?

☐ About right
☐ Too hot
■ Too cold

Figure 3.1   Pie chart showing answers to a question on a survey of patient satisfaction with catering facilities.

What proportion of respondents gave each of the three answers?

Study 2

Figure 3.2 shows the prices for 4 weeks of treatment for seven different drugs, each at the appropriate dose for the same complaint.

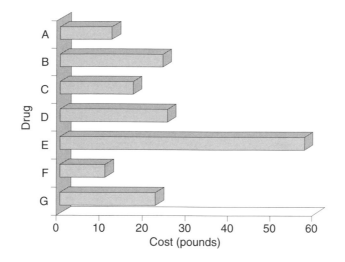

Figure 3.2   Bar chart showing costs of seven different drugs.

Which are the cheapest and most expensive drugs, and what are their respective costs?

Study 3

A GP's surgery keeps track of the number of missed appointments with the doctor each week. Figure 3.3 shows a plot of the data for an 8-week period.

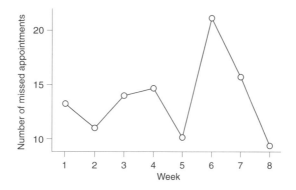

Figure 3.3   Plot showing numbers of missed appointments at a GP's surgery over an 8-week period.

What happened in week 6?

Study 4

A therapist is interested in how her client base has changed over time. She looks back at her records and counts how many clients she has had over the past few years. Figure 3.4 shows a plot of the resulting data.

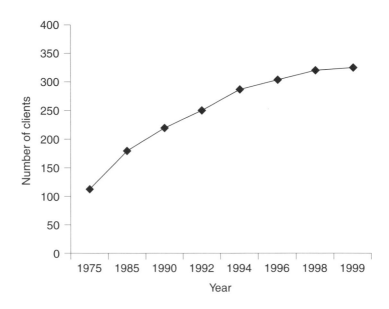

Figure 3.4   Plot of number of clients against year in which records were inspected.

Over which period was there the greatest rate of increase in the number of her clients?

Figures 3.5 to 3.8 show alternative versions of these four charts. Which of the charts do you find easiest to interpret, and how do your answers vary?

Pie charts

Figures 3.1 and 3.5 are examples of pie charts. The chart is a circle divided into slices, where the size of each slice is proportional to the number represented. Here the charts show the proportions of replies to each of the three different response options. For a pie chart to be meaningful, the whole area

Question: What is your opinion of the temperature of the cooked food?

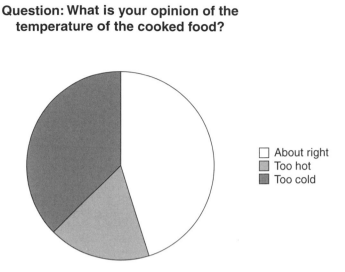

Figure 3.5 Two-dimensional pie chart showing answers to a question on a survey of patient satisfaction with catering facilities.

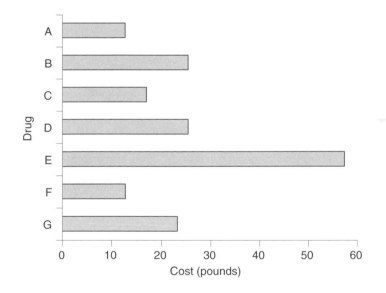

Figure 3.6 Two-dimensional bar chart showing costs of seven different drugs.

must mean something. In this case the whole area represents the whole set of replies. (Note that it does not necessarily represent the answers from all in-patients at the time of the survey. Some people may not have completed a questionnaire, or may have failed to answer this question.) In fact, 36% of

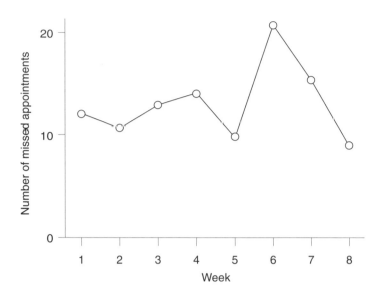

Figure 3.7   Plot showing numbers of missed appointments at a GP's surgery over an 8-week period. The vertical axis starts at zero.

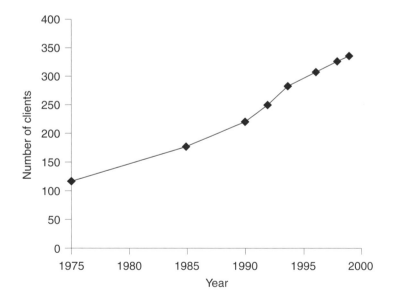

Figure 3.8   Plot of number of clients against year in which records were inspected. The horizontal axis has a uniform scale.

respondents said that the food was 'too cold', 45% replied that it was 'about right', and the remaining 19% said that the food was 'too hot'.

The perspective effect in Figure 3.1 makes the chart eye-catching. However, most people find that this also makes it more difficult to interpret than the flat two-dimensional chart shown in Figure 3.5. The three-dimensional chart shows volume as opposed to area. Often the volume of the slice nearer the front appears disproportionately larger and those at the back appear disproportionately smaller. How did you fare?

Pie charts are useful for displaying nominal or ordinal data, where the components are part of a whole. They are not very common in scientific papers, but there is a proliferation of them in advertising material and glossy reports. Sadly, the three-dimensional charts are very prevalent.

The pie-chart slices are often labelled with the percentages that they represent. This is good practice, but the visual impression of the picture is still stronger for most people, and you need to discipline yourself to look at the numbers and not just the apparent areas or volumes.

Even if the pie chart displays the percentage figures, there is still a loss of information from the original data. We do not know how many people answered the question, or what proportion of the in-patients this represents. Moreover, we know nothing about the profiles of the people who gave each answer, or about any relationships between the answers to this question and the answers to other questions in the survey.

Bar charts

The three-dimensional problem also affects Figure 3.2, which is an example of a bar chart. Drug F is the cheapest at £12.87, while drug E is the most expensive at £57.08. These are examples of horizontal bar charts. Bar charts can be horizontal or vertical. The bars should be labelled (in this case with the drug labels A to F), and the length or height of the bar is proportional to the statistic of interest, which in this case is cost. Although it is relatively easy to *rank* the bars in size on either chart, most people find it easier to read the *actual* values from the two-dimensional chart. As with the pie charts, the visual impression of the picture is often stronger, even if the bars are labelled with the actual data values.

It is always important to read the labels and text that accompany any such chart.

Time-series plots

Figures 3.3 and 3.7 show examples of time-series plots. The data are measured over time, and each point represents the value for a particular week. Since there is a logical order to the points, they can be joined up. The major difference between the two charts is the scale on the vertical axis. In Figure 3.3 this starts above zero, whereas in Figure 3.7 it starts at zero. The overall effect is that in Figure 3.3 the fluctuations tend to be exaggerated. Unless you look carefully at the vertical scale, it appears as if the number of missed appointments at week 6 is more than twice the normal typical value. In fact, the number is 22 compared to an average of about 13. The 'jump' is less pronounced in Figure 3.7. Graphs like this can be made to look quite different by 'zooming in' or 'zooming out'. It is not always sensible to start a scale at zero. For example, if you did this with patients' temperature charts, all you would do is waste a lot of paper at the bottom of the graph. However, the range of normal values on a temperature chart is well understood, and such a chart is not open to misinterpretation. This is not the case for graphs in general. The lesson is clear – make sure that you look at the scales.

Figure 3.4 is even more bizarre. Did you notice that the scale on the horizontal axis is not uniform? It is labelled by the years whose records have been inspected. However, these values were not measured at equal intervals. This makes the graph extremely difficult to interpret. The visual impression gained from Figure 3.4 is that the rate of growth in client numbers is highest early on. In fact it is clear from Figure 3.8 that the highest rate of growth is between 1990 and 1995. Graphs like this should not appear at all, but this one is included here for two reasons. First, it is a warning about the way in which poor graphs can distort data. Second, a graph like this was recently submitted to a healthcare journal (but not accepted). Be warned.

Scatter plots

A scatter plot is used to show the relationship between a pair of variables. These are usually both continuous variables. Figure 3.9 shows an example of a scatter plot. The data are from 30 children treated for excessive overjet (malocclusion) – that is, front teeth sticking out. Each point, denoted by a circle, shows the change in upper incisor angle (in degrees) on the vertical axis plotted against the upper incisor angle (in degrees) before treatment. For most of the children the upper incisor angle decreases during treatment. With one exception, the values on the vertical axis are negative, and many are greater than 10 degrees in size. Moreover, children with larger upper incisor angles before treatment tend to show the largest changes in upper incisor angle. Thus there seems to be a relationship between the two variables, but it is not very strong. The symbols form a 'scatter' because, unlike the case with the data in the time-series plot, there is no logical reason to join them up.

Sometimes both variables arise 'on the same footing'. More often one variable is 'dependent' on the other. The *dependent* variable is then represented on the

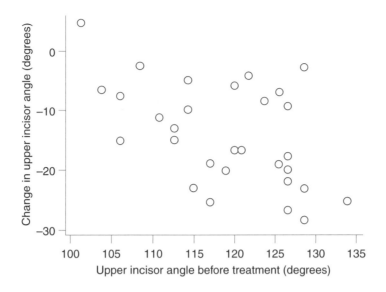

Figure 3.9 Scatter plot showing relationship between the change in upper incisor angle plotted against the upper incisor angle before treatment for 30 children treated for malocclusion.

vertical axis. Typically, if one variable influences another then the influencing variable is represented on the horizontal axis. In an experimental situation, where the experimenter has control over one of the variables, this variable is represented on the horizontal axis. The common terminology is *predictor variable* to denote the variable controlled by the experimenter, and *response variable* to denote the other variable. In the example shown in Figure 3.9, one would expect that the change in upper incisor angle might be influenced by its initial value, so the choice of which variable goes on which axis is as shown.

Multiple and component bar charts

Table 3.1 shows data collected from 18 patients attending a therapist's clinic. These patients were questioned about a number of complaints, and were asked whether they had suffered them during the previous couple of weeks, in the past but not in the previous couple of weeks, or not at all. Data for three of the complaints are given here. These data can be represented by a variety of bar charts, and examples are given in Figures 3.10 to 3.13.

Figure 3.10 is a multiple bar chart, which shows the frequency of each reply for each complaint on the same chart. By comparing the bars you are able to compare the numbers of responses for each complaint and to make comparisons between complaints. The chart contains all of the information

Table 3.1   Data describing 18 patients' experiences of three complaints

Complaint	Suffered in the previous 2 weeks	Suffered in the past	Never experienced
Migraine	3	4	11
Sinusitis	1	1	16
Lower back pain	2	5	11

from Table 3.1. Figure 3.11 is like a multiple pie chart. It depicts the proportions of answers for each condition, but not the actual numbers. Using this chart it is much easier to compare the proportions, but not the actual numbers, of people who have chosen each answer for each complaint. Figures 3.12 and 3.13 represent the data from positive responses only (i.e. omitting patients who had no experience of the complaint). Figure 3.12 shows the breakdown of actual responses, and Figure 3.13 shows the data as percentages. Thus it is clear in Figure 3.12, but not in Figure 3.13, that few people have experienced sinusitis, and that equal numbers have suffered migraine and lower back pain. A possible danger with Figure 3.13 is that the percentages are based on very small numbers. For example, there were only two positive responses to sinusitis, so the figure of 50% who have experienced it recently could be quite misleading. Therefore it is good practice to label each bar with its total frequency, as well as the component percentages, in charts like Figures 3.11 and 3.13.

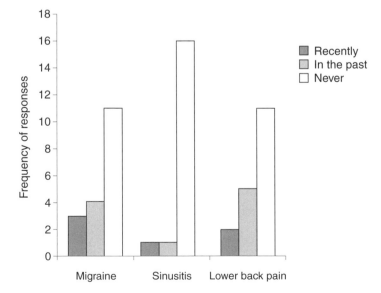

Figure 3.10   Multiple bar chart showing 18 patients' experiences of three complaints.

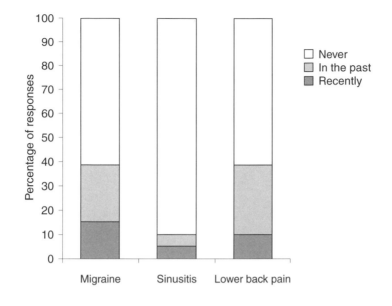

Figure 3.11   Percentage component bar chart showing proportions of responses describing 18 patients' experiences of three complaints.

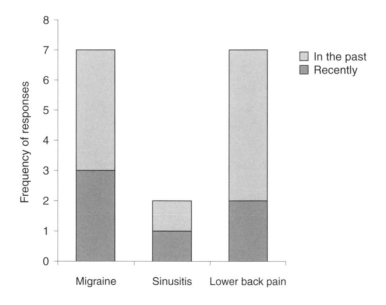

Figure 3.12   Component bar chart showing 18 patients' experiences of three complaints.

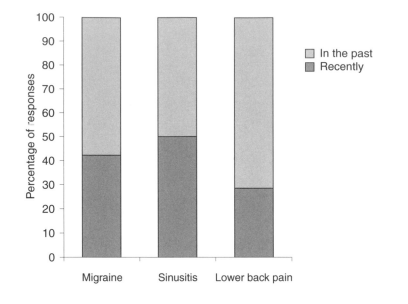

Figure 3.13 Percentage component bar chart showing 18 patients' experiences of three complaints.

The charts have many similarities, but they emphasise different aspects of the data. Which one is 'best' will depend on the features that you are trying to communicate. When interpreting such data you should look carefully at the type of chart that is being used. Do not jump to conclusions without checking exactly what is being displayed. Furthermore, you should have the confidence to ask questions about the data.

Histograms

Histograms look very like bar charts, but they are essentially different. Histograms are used to show the distributions of continuous variables. Table 3.2 shows the ages of the 18 patients attending the therapist's clinic. Age is really a continuous variable, but the values are recorded here as whole numbers. In order to create a histogram the data are grouped into classes (e.g. less than 40, at least 40 but less than 50, etc.). Bars are drawn above the corresponding intervals such that the *area* of the bar is proportional to the number of values in that class. There should be no gaps between the bars. Most commonly the classes are of equal width, so the heights are proportional to these values, but this is not always the case. Figures 3.14 to 3.16 show three

Table 3.2 Ages (in years) of the 18 patients attending the therapist's clinic

58 62 41 53 52 38 48 46 28 56 65 68 45 45 51 60 56 58

histograms depicting the data from Table 3.2. Note how they appear slightly different. This is because of the different choice of class boundaries in each case. Histograms can be very useful for giving a general idea of the distribution of values, but they are very sensitive to the choice of classes. For this reason they should be interpreted with care unless they are based on a large sample.

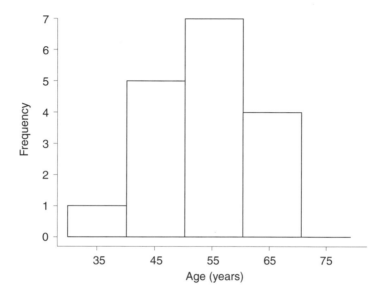

Figure 3.14   Histogram showing the ages in years of the 18 patients.

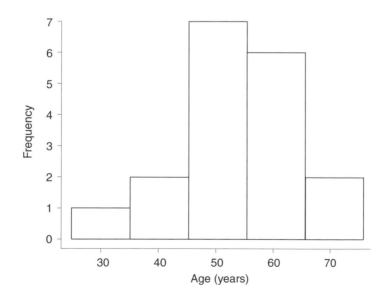

Figure 3.15   Histogram showing the ages in years of the 18 patients.

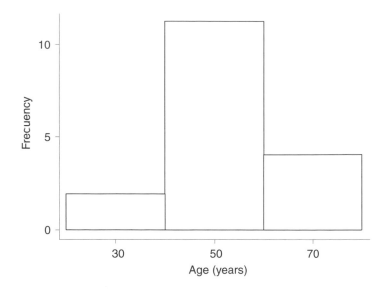

Figure 3.16   Histogram showing the ages in years of the 18 patients.

What to look for

Lies are perpetrated by a chart that gives a misleading picture of an effect. In a comprehensive and very readable book about pictorial representation,[1] Tufte defines a 'lie factor' as follows:

$$\text{lie factor} = \frac{\text{size of apparent effect}}{\text{size of actual effect}}.$$

A lie factor of 1 is fair. Large or small values of a lie factor mean that you are in danger of being misled. Duff[2] also gives some interesting examples of chart misuse. Here is a list of things to look out for:

- shapes or pictures not drawn to scale
- unnecessary use of perspective or an extra dimension
- no title/information about the source of the data
- axes not labelled
- scale unclear
- scale not uniform
- vertical scale not starting at zero.

Final warning

Finally, in order to drive the point home, consider Figures 3.17 to 3.20, which show the same set of data in time-series plots, where the scales are the same but the aspect ratios of the graphs differ – that is, the degree of squareness varies. Notice how the overall impression varies. Graphs which artificially inflate an effect are often called 'gee-whiz' graphs. If you see an apparently exciting feature in a graph you should double-check that you have interpreted it correctly.

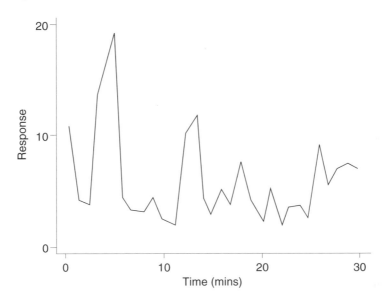

Figure 3.17   Time-series plot.

The content of this chapter is not merely academic. A paper in the *British Medical Journal* showed how the method of data display can affect physicians' decisions and have potentially far-reaching consequences.[3] The accompanying editorial[4] stated that:

> the format in which information is presented significantly influences clinical decisions, ranging from the accuracy of obstetric judgements to the speed of interpreting laboratory tests or intensive-care data. As shown vividly by pharmaceutical advertisements, the potential for influencing doctors' decisions by changing the format of information extends beyond the choice of graphics to the statistics used to describe trial results and how options are worded, such as 'chances of survival' versus 'chances of death'.

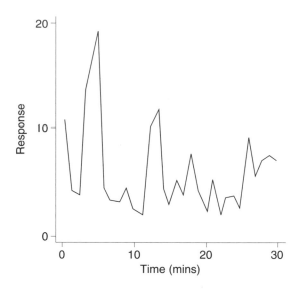

Figure 3.18   Time-series plot of the data shown in Figure 3.17.

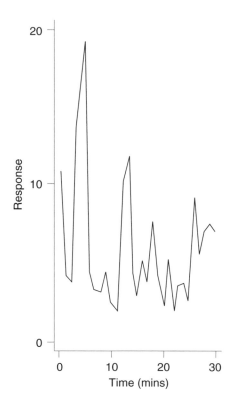

Figure 3.19   Time-series plot of the data shown in Figure 3.17.

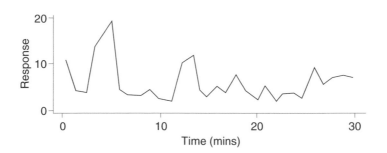

Figure 3.20   Time-series plot of the data shown in Figure 3.17.

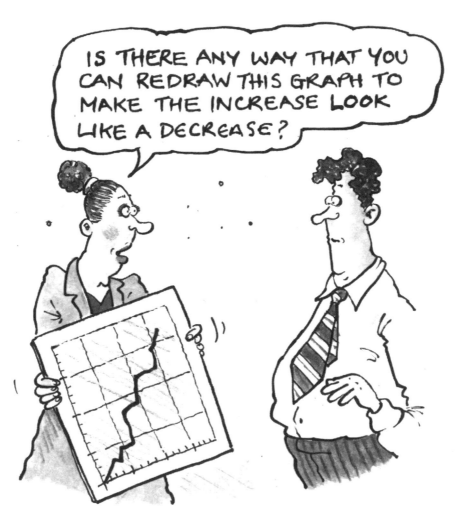

Summary

Graphs and charts are very good methods of displaying summaries of data. However, they are open to misuse and misinterpretation. Always ask the following questions.

- What is the chart supposed to show?
- Where did the data come from?
- What was the sample size?

In addition, always look at the following:

- the caption
- the accompanying text
- labels
- the scales of the axes
- the keys for the interpretation of shading.

Beware of 'gee-whiz' factors – always double-check that you have interpreted the chart correctly.

CHAPTER FOUR

It's a mean old scene

Although charts and graphs are useful, numerical summaries of data are more important. Sizes of effects and strengths of association need to be quantified. Numbers that summarise key features of data are called *summary statistics*. Again, the key skill is to use a set of summary statistics that adequately and fairly summarise the data. This chapter therefore explores the commonly used summary statistics. The ideas are introduced via the results of research into the possible effects of a television drama on suicidal behaviour[1] (Case Study D). At the end you should be able to:

- interpret a variety of summary statistics
- describe the situations in which different summary statistics are valid
- distinguish between symmetrical and skewed data.

Scene setting

Researchers have argued about the effects that television drama programmes might have on the suicidal behaviour of vulnerable people. In 1996, the UK television drama *Casualty* ran an episode in which a pilot took a serious overdose of paracetamol. The fact that this episode was given advance publicity meant that a group of researchers was able to conduct a prospective study of the effects of that particular episode. A total of 49 hospitals collected data. They supplied weekly data about all of the individuals who presented with overdose during the 3 weeks before the broadcast or during the 3 weeks afterwards. During this period clinicians in general psychiatric services were asked to return questionnaires with details obtained from the assessment of the patients. In total, 25 of the 49 hospitals returned questionnaires for a total of 1047 patients. The statistical analysis was quite complicated, but basically compared the presentation rates before the broadcast with the values obtained afterwards. During the 3 weeks before the broadcast a total of 2127 patients presented at the hospitals. In the 3 weeks after the broadcast the number of presenting patients was 2276, with a marked increase in the week immediately following the programme. The paper reporting the study contains several tables of summary statistics.

Table 4.1 shows some of the reported statistics from the questionnaire responses. Note that the notation '$n =$' is a shorthand for 'the number of values (responses, subjects, patients, etc.) was'.

Table 4.1   Some summary statistics from the study about suicide attempts; unless otherwise stated, values are counts (with percentages shown in parentheses)

	3 weeks before broadcast			3 weeks after broadcast		
	Third week	Second week	First week	First week	Second week	Third week
Number of patients	187	190	186	194	163	127
Median age (and range) in years	31 (12–90)	29 (13–83)	31 (12–89)	30 (13–70)	30 (7–82)	27.5 (13–82)
Opinions among those who watched most recent episode of *Casualty*	$n = 22$	$n = 23$	$n = 26$	$n = 32$	$n = 23$	$n = 14$
General TV viewing influenced choice of drug	1 (5)	2 (9)	1 (4)	3 (10)	4 (17)	3 (21)
Index episode influenced decision to take overdose				6 (20)	2 (9)	2 (14)
Index episode influenced choice of drug				5 (17)	3 (13)	2 (14)
Index episode influenced speed of seeking help				3 (10)	1 (5)	3 (21)

The table shows both counts and percentages. This is good practice. For the questions about the influence of television, it is the *percentages* that are of most interest when comparing the weeks. However, as was discussed in Chapter 3, percentages can be very sensitive to the totals from which they are calculated. For example, consider the apparent difference in those who admit to being influenced by television in weeks 1 and 2 after the programme. These values are 10% and 17%, respectively. Closer inspection of the data shows that these are supposedly calculated from 3/32 and 4/23 subjects. Had the numbers been slightly different, at 4/32 and 3/23, the corresponding percentages would have been 12.5% and 13%, respectively. The second percentage value is still higher, but the difference is far less striking. Therefore presenting the percentages without the raw counts would have been potentially misleading.

It can also be misleading to present counts without percentages. For example, among those patients who presented after the broadcast and who said that they had watched the most recent episode of *Casualty*, ten admitted to being influenced in their choice of drug by general television viewing. The corresponding number before the broadcast was four. This looks interesting. However, there were more presentations of suicide attempts after the broadcast, and this may distort the numbers. Percentages should therefore be compared. As the paper states, '*Casualty* viewers attending after the episode were slightly more likely to state that general television viewing influenced their choice of drug than those attending before the broadcast (14% vs. 6% ...)'. These percentage values are computed from 10/69 and 4/71 patients, respectively. In this particular example the total numbers of responses for watchers of *Casualty* before and after the broadcast were similar. Notice how important it is to use the correct number for the total (the number on the 'bottom' of the ratio) when calculating the percentage. Here it is the number of respondents who said that they had watched *Casualty*. While it is obviously possible to calculate percentages from counts, most people find it difficult to do this for several figures and then to compare them in their heads. This is why it is good practice for counts and percentages to be presented if both are of potential interest.

The moral should be clear. Beware of counts or percentages that are presented in isolation. If you encounter a table containing one and not the other, try to compute the missing statistics. If you have insufficient information to be able to do this, you may have good reason to suspect that you are being deceived, or at least to doubt the quality of the study.

Below are some examples of unfair statements. What else would you want to know before answering the associated question?

In a study comparing drug X with drug Y, 50% more patients reported the side-effect of nausea with drug X than with drug Y.

Which drug has the worst side-effects profile?

In the past 12 months five people died in the operating-theatre at hospital A while undergoing T; over the same period the number who died in hospital B, only 20 miles away, was only one.

Which hospital has the more favourable record?

Much more contextual information would be needed in practice. For example, in the first question, how effective were the two drugs, and what other side-effects were recorded? All other things being equal, it is still important to know *how many subjects* there were in each treatment group and *how many actual reported cases of nausea*.

Suppose that there were 50 patients in each group, and two taking drug Y reported nausea. How would you feel about the relative merits of the drugs? How would your answer change if the number in each group was 100, and 60 patients taking drug Y reported nausea?

In the second example a lot of contextual information is missing. Were the groups of patients at each hospital similar in terms of, for example, severity of clinical problem and age profile? Assuming that they were comparable in all respects, consider the following two scenarios. First, 50 operations were performed at hospital A and 10 operations at hospital B. Second, there were 100 operations at hospital A and 200 operations at hospital B. You probably feel quite differently about the relative safety at the hospitals for these two scenarios. People without scruples can try to influence your beliefs by the way in which they present partial information. Be on your guard.

Mean

In the study of suicide attempts the participating hospitals were classified by geographical region of the country. One of the background statistics collected was the number of annual new attendances at Accident and Emergency departments for each hospital. The numbers are counts, and they are examples of discrete data. The average for each region was presented. For example, there were three participating hospitals in Scotland, and the average for these three hospitals was 59 040. The average for the four participating hospitals in the West Midlands was higher, at 76 800. The value 59 040 was computed by adding together the three values for the hospitals and dividing by three. This is what people generally understand by an *average*. The technical term is the *mean*. In fact, in statistics there are different types of average, and the term mean denotes a particular type. The mean is used as a typical 'middle of the road' sort of value. Some values will be greater than the mean, but on average these will be balanced out by about the same number of values being less than the mean.

Median

Unfortunately, the 'middle of the road' notion does not always apply to the mean. It is fine if the data are symmetrical (in fact, there are some symmetrical distributions for which the mean is not very useful, but these do not often arise in medical data). In symmetrical data, for every large value you expect to get a small value the same distance away from the mean in the opposite direction. However, not all data are like this.

For example, in the questionnaires the researchers asked how long the delay was between the patient taking the drug and subsequently seeking advice. Table 4.2 shows some of the data describing the responses for patients who took a paracetamol compound, who said that they were not viewers of *Casualty* and who presented during the 3 weeks before the broadcast.

Table 4.2   Summary of responses from 188 (out of 193) of the patients presenting 3 weeks before the broadcast who were non-viewers of *Casualty*, and who took a substance containing paracetamol

Delay between paracetamol overdose and presentation (hours)	Number (percentage)
<6	139 (74)
6–12	23 (12)
>12	26 (14)

Delay times are positive continuous values, but the reported data are grouped into ordinal classes. From these coded data it is fairly clear that the values are not symmetrical. Most of the responses (139/188) are in the 'less than 6 hours' class. A moderate number (23/188) are in the '6–12 hours' class, and a similar number are in the 'more than 12 hours' class. Similar patterns occurred for the non-viewers after the episode, and also for the viewers before and after the episode. Most of the people who took a paracetamol substance sought help within less than 6 hours, about one-eighth waited for up to 12 hours, and approximately one-eighth waited for more than 12 hours. Data shaped like this are described as *skewed*, as opposed to *symmetrical*. In this case there is a clump of low values together with some medium values and some high values. Given the actual values for each patient, it would be possible to calculate the mean, but this would not be a 'middle of the road' value. The long delay times would tend to make the mean value large, so that *more than half* of the values would lie below the mean. For data like this a better 'middle of the road' value is the actual *middle* value when the data are arranged in increasing order. In other words, it is the value at which half the data values are below it and half are above it – you cannot get much more 'middle of the road' than that! This summary statistic is called the *median.* For symmetrical data the mean and the median are about equal. You might wonder why the mean is used at all, in that case. The reason is that the mathematical properties of the mean are better from a theoretical point of view, and therefore the more efficient statistical methods can be used for the mean. Some of these ideas are discussed in the next chapter, but the underlying theory is well beyond the scope of this book.

   In the above study the ages of patients were recorded. Ages are positive continuous values, but they appear to have been recorded as whole numbers. The summary statistics are shown in Table 4.1. The data do appear skewed. For example, the range of ages in the first week of the study (the third week before the broadcast) is 12 to 90 years, but the median is 31 years. A similar pattern exists for the other weeks. This means that half of the patients were aged between 12 and 31 years, and half of them were aged between 31 and 90 years. The data are skewed in the same direction as those in Table 4.2. The researchers are therefore correct in reporting medians rather than means, as the latter would tend to be disproportionately high.

Variability

In addition to quoting the mean or median, the researchers also report the *range* of values for the patients' ages and the number of annual new attendances at the hospitals. The range is defined by the smallest and largest values in the data. It is informative because the mean or median on its own gives an inadequate description of a set of data. Figures 4.1 and 4.2 show two samples of size 50 from symmetrical distributions with means of 20. The histograms are both approximately symmetrical about the value 20. You may not think that they look very symmetrical, but such deviations from symmetry are natural for samples of size 50. However, if you look at the horizontal scale (remember Chapter 2), you will see that the range of values in Figure 4.2 is much greater. The data in Figure 4.1 are much more tightly clustered around the mean. In other words, the variability or spread changes from one sample to the other. In the first sample, the values range from 16 to 24, with the middle 25 values (50%) lying between 18 and 22. For the second sample, the values range from 9 to 31, and the middle 25 values (50%) lie between 16 and 24. However, it is impossible to see this level of detail in the histograms. Spread (or variability) is fundamental to statistical methodology – no variability

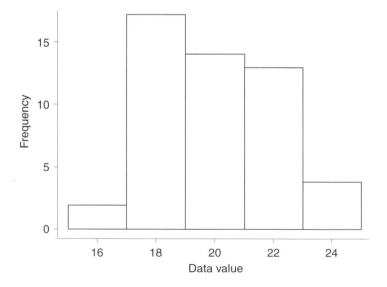

Figure 4.1   Histogram of a sample of size 50 from a symmetrical distribution with a mean of 20.

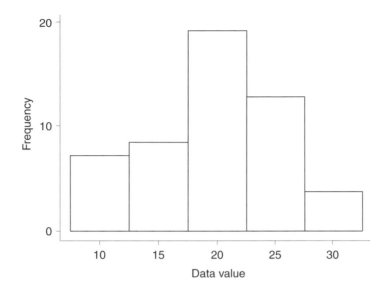

Figure 4.2 Histogram of a sample of size 50 from a symmetrical distribution with a mean of 20. The spread of values is greater than that shown in Figure 4.1.

would mean no need for statistics. It should be clear from these examples why a measure of spread can be extremely important. In some situations you might prefer a variable which had a slightly less favourable mean but a smaller spread. This is because you could easily obtain values far removed from the mean when the spread is high. High spread means low predictability.

For symmetrically shaped data, especially data such as those shown in Figures 4.1 and 4.2, the measure of spread that is paired with the mean is called the *standard deviation*. You will be spared the formula, but this statistic essentially gives an average distance of the set of values from their mean. For data like these (for more details, *see* Chapter 5) the following rules of thumb apply:

- 68% of values lie within one standard deviation of the mean
- 95% of values lie within two standard deviations of the mean
- over 99% of values lie within three standard deviations of the mean.

The *variance* is the *standard deviation squared*. If the standard deviation is 2, then the variance is 4. The standard deviation is much easier to interpret, but you may find people referring to the variance.

For skewed data the mean is not generally useful, so measures of distance from the mean are fairly useless. The standard deviation is therefore not a natural partner for the median. The measures that are used capture the ideas of the rules of thumb given above. For example, find the value below which 25% of the values lie, and the value above which 25% lie. These are called the *lower quartile* and *upper quartile*, respectively. Then the middle half of the data will lie between the lower and upper quartiles. In fact:

- 25% of values lie below the lower quartile
- 25% of values lie between the lower quartile and the median
- 25% of values lie between the median and the upper quartile
- 25% of values lie above the upper quartile.

So instead of the standard deviation, the *inter-quartile range* is used. This is the difference between the lower and upper quartiles. It can be quoted as a single number, but more often the two quartiles are stated.

These concepts are illustrated in Figures 4.3 and 4.4, which show two samples of skewed data. The summary statistics are shown in Table 4.3.

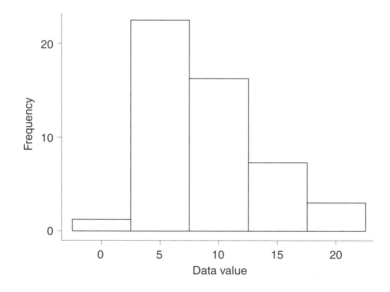

Figure 4.3   Histogram of a sample of size 50 from a right-skewed distribution.

It is worth noting that the means for these two samples are 8.4 and 12.6, respectively. Note that the means are larger than the medians, due to the influence of the large values in the right-hand tail of the histograms. This effect is particularly pronounced for the second set of data. When the histograms are skewed in this way with a long right-hand tail they are described as *right-skewed*. When the tail is on the left-hand side they are described as *left-skewed*.

The quartiles (divisions into quarters) are examples of *percentiles* – that is, divisions into hundredths. The lower quartile is the 25th percentile, and the median is the 50th percentile. You can use the 10th, 90th, 75th or any other percentile, as long as it makes clinical sense.

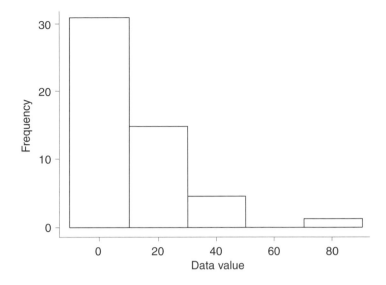

Figure 4.4 Histogram of a sample of size 50 from a right-skewed distribution. Skewness is very evident.

Table 4.3 Summary statistics for the data in the histograms shown in Figures 4.3 and 4.4

Data source	Minimum	Lower quartile	Median	Upper quartile	Maximum
Figure 4.3	2	5	7	10	19
Figure 4.4	1	4	8	15	76

Rounding

You should always look at the accuracy of data. Ideally, researchers should quote the accuracy of their reported data. Do not be fooled by data that appear to be extremely precise, especially if you doubt that they could have been measured to that level of accuracy. Furthermore, computed statistics cannot be more accurate than the data from which they were calculated. Summary statistics such as the mean and standard deviation might require one more decimal place than the original data, but not several.

For example, the mean of the following data

$$2 \quad 5 \quad 7 \quad 8 \quad 9 \quad 12$$

is 43/6, which is 7.1666. It could be quoted as 7.2, or possibly as 7, depending on the intended use, but no more than one decimal place should be quoted.

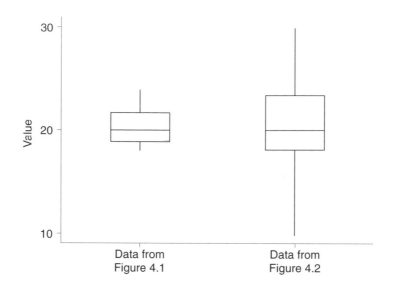

Figure 4.5 Boxplots of the symmetrical data in the histograms shown in Figures 4.1 and 4.2.

More charts – boxplots

Chapter 2 described several charts and plots. Now that you know about medians and quartiles, there is another plot you should know about – a boxplot. Examples of boxplots are given in Figure 4.5. A boxplot consists of a vertical or horizontal box with lines extending outward from the sides of the box. The lower or left-hand side of the box is the lower quartile, and the upper or right-hand side of the box is the upper quartile. The line dividing the box (which is not necessarily in the middle of the box) is the median. The lines extending outward from the box are known as 'whiskers', and they extend to the minimum and maximum values, provided that they are not a long way from the box. If there are values that are a long way from the bulk of the data, these are viewed as unusual, and are often denoted by asterisks. Their technical name is *outliers.*

Figure 4.5 shows the data from the histograms illustrated in Figures 4.1 and 4.2 represented in vertical boxplots on the same scale. Boxplots are particularly useful for comparing sets of data in this way. The plots are fairly symmetrical, with the median line near the middle of the box. The plot for the data with greater spread is more elongated. No outliers are marked. The horizontal boxplots in Figure 4.6 represent the data from the two skewed histograms. The plots are not symmetrical and there are outliers. The whiskers on the right-hand side are longer than those on the left-hand side, and the median is closer to the lower quartile than to the upper quartile. These characteristics of skewness are very evident for the data from Figure 4.4.

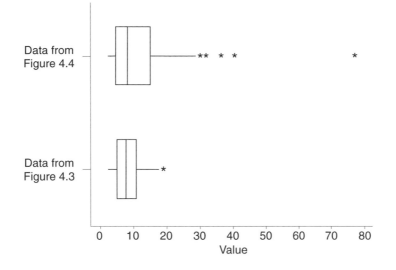

Figure 4.6 Boxplots of the right-skewed data in the histograms shown in Figures 4.3 and 4.4.

As with histograms, you should not take too much notice of the details of a boxplot from a small sample. However, for moderate to large samples boxplots are good methods, both for investigating skewness of data and for comparing two or more sets of data. In fact, for small sets of data the quartiles are not very useful, and it is better to quote the range instead.

Some more illustrative examples are given below.

Study of a nurse consultation system

There is increasing pressure on UK general practitioners, especially with regard to demand for out-of-hours care. One solution is to operate a nurse consultation system out of hours. A randomised controlled trial was conducted in Wiltshire to determine the safety of such a service[2] (Case Study A). The design of the study was, appropriately, fairly complicated. During the study the service that was offered alternated randomly between normal service and service with a nurse telephone consultation. Prior to their telephone call, patients did not know which service was on offer. The researchers logged the number and management of calls for each service, and the study design enabled these statistics to be calculated for weekly periods. The aim was to determine whether there was an *equivalent* number of adverse events in the two regimes.

One objective of the research was to establish how the calls that were received were managed. Table 4.4 shows the summary statistics relevant to this question. The total numbers of calls received for each service were similar, but the table shows a breakdown of the management outcome of the calls,

Table 4.4 Management outcome of calls during the study; numbers of calls are shown (with percentages in parentheses)

Management outcome	Usual service (n = 7308)	Nurse telephone consultation (n = 7184)
Calls managed with nurse telephone advice	–	3581 (50)
Calls managed with telephone advice from GP	3629 (50)	1109 (15)
Patient attended primary care centre	1934 (26)	1177 (16)
Patient was visited at home by GP	1745 (24)	1317 (18)

giving both counts and percentages. This enables comparisons to be made. Thus for the normal service half of the calls were managed with telephone advice from the general practitioner. While the nurse consultation system was in operation the nurses were able to deal with half of the calls. There were corresponding decreases in the proportion of calls that used general practitioner advice on the telephone, or required the patient to visit the primary care centre, or required the general practitioner to visit the patient at home. The greatest reduction was in the number of calls handled by the general practitioner. The fact that numbers and percentages are both given enables these comparisons to be made easily and with confidence. Since the data were collected for weekly periods, it was possible to give more detailed analyses of weekly statistics. A summary is shown in Table 4.5. The statistics give an idea of the weekly number of calls that can be handled, and the effects in terms of a reduction in workload for the general practitioner.

Table 4.5 Management outcome of calls, comparing calls received in weeks during the study; median values are shown (with interquartile range in parentheses)

Management outcome	Usual service	Nurse telephone consultation
Calls managed with nurse telephone advice	–	138 (121–143)
Calls managed with telephone advice from GP	132 (119–148)	36 (31–57)
Patient attended primary care centre	68 (58–79)	40 (35–50)
Patient was visited at home by GP	66 (57–76)	49 (44–60)

The summary statistics given are the median and interquartile range. Examination of these statistics suggests that the data from the period when the nurse consultation service operated are skewed. During these periods the median number of calls in a weekly period managed by the nurse telephone advice was 138. The interquartile range was 121 to 143. The 'box' part of the boxplot for these data is shown in Figure 4.7. Thus 25% of the weekly periods had between 121 and 138 calls managed by the nurses, and a further

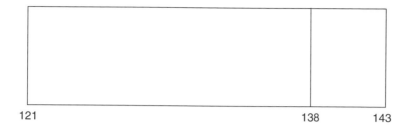

Figure 4.7   Box showing median and upper and lower quartiles for the calls managed with nurse telephone advice.

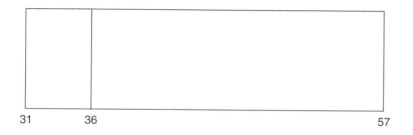

Figure 4.8   Box showing median and quartiles for the calls managed by telephone advice from the GP when the nurse telephone consultation system was in operation.

25% had between 138 and 143 calls managed by the nurses. These data are *negatively skewed* – for most weekly periods the number is high, but there are some weeks for which it is low. Figure 4.8 shows the box for the data about calls that were managed by telephone advice from the GP, when the nurses were available. These data are *positively skewed* – there is a group of low numbers (25% of the weeks have between 31 and 36 calls handled in this way) and a small number of weeks with large numbers. The researchers are therefore being fair in presenting medians and interquartile ranges. They have chosen the interquartile range in preference to the range. Researchers often do this because the range is influenced by extreme outliers and by the number of data values collected. If there is one very large and one very small outlier, these will define the range, but they may not be typical of the bulk of the data. The quartiles, which define the middle half of the data values, are not so sensitive to extreme values, and are useful provided that the data set is not small.

Study of eating disorders in adolescent girls

A group of researchers in Canada set out to compare the prevalence of eating disorders in adolescent girls with type I diabetes with that in their non-diabetic peers[3] (Case Study F). Subjects with diabetes were recruited from three hospitals, and the comparison group (*control group*) was recruited from schools. The sampling was designed to ensure that there were approximately three times as many non-diabetics as diabetics, and that the profiles with regard to age and site were similar in the two groups. The paper presented a table of demographic data describing the girls who took part in the study. Some of these data are shown in Table 4.6.

Table 4.6   Some demographic features of subjects in the study; mean values are shown (with standard deviation in parentheses)

Characteristic	Diabetic girls (n = 361)	Non-diabetic girls (n = 1114)
Age (years)	14.9 (2.0)	14.8 (1.9)
Body mass index	22.7 (3.8)	20.6 (3.3)
Age at onset of diabetes (years)	8.1 (3.6)	–
Duration of diabetes (years)	6.7 (3.6)	–

Here the authors have chosen the mean and standard deviation as summary statistics. This is what many researchers do, sometimes seemingly without much thought about the appropriateness of these values. Here the data may well be symmetrical, and the choice of summary statistics is appropriate. However, there is some evidence that the data about the duration of diabetes might be slightly skewed. As was stated earlier, for symmetrically-shaped data over 95% of the values lie within two standard deviations of the mean. The mean and standard deviation for the duration are 6.7 and 3.6 years, respectively. The above rule would translate into 'over 95% of values lie between –0.5 years and 13.9 years'. However, a duration must be positive, so the lowest value must be zero. Therefore there is a slight hint that the data might be skewed. Here it is probably not a serious problem. However, if you ever see data for a variable which you know is always greater than zero and for which the mean is much less than twice the standard deviation, you can conclude that the data are skewed and that inappropriate summary statistics are being used.

   For example, look back at the histogram of skewed data shown in Figure 4.4. The mean and standard deviation for these data are 12.6 and 13.3, respectively. If you knew that all of the values had to be greater than zero, you would know that the data were skewed by the fact that the mean is smaller than the standard deviation. For these data the mean and standard deviation are poor summary statistics. The median and interquartile range (as quoted earlier) are much more meaningful.

What about other types of data?

The data considered so far in this chapter have been continuous or at least discrete. Because ordinal data have a natural order, you can use the median and either the interquartile range or the range to describe them. Some ordinal variables (e.g. stage of cancer) do not behave much like continuous variables. However, others may share many characteristics of the symmetrical data illustrated in Figures 4.1 and 4.2. Examples would include scores for quality of life or disability. Strictly speaking these are ordinal, but during validation of the score it may have been established that they behave very like continuous symmetrical variables. If this is the case, they can be summarised by the mean and standard deviation. However, it is important to be wary. If people treat ordinal data as if they were continuous without providing a reasoned justification for this, you may have cause to be sceptical about what they have done.

Means, standard deviations, medians, ranges and quartiles can *never* be used for nominal data. You may be able to press the computer keys and get a number for, say, the mean of patients' religion, but it would be of no use. For nominal data, if there is one class which occurs more than the others then this is defined as the *mode*. The mode is a suitable summary statistic for such data. However, this is often inadequate. One reason is that the mode alone gives no idea of the variability in the data. There is no simple statistic describing the variability in nominal data, and frequencies and percentages are often the best summaries.

Tables 4.7 and 4.8 show two sets of nominal data describing marital status. In each case the mode is the class 'living alone', because it has the highest number of responses. This is possibly useful for the data in Table 4.7, but not for the data in Table 4.8. In Table 4.8 there are three classes with approximately equal numbers of responses, and a fourth class with a lower number of responses. Common sense should not be abandoned when summarising data.

Table 4.7 Nominal data describing marital status

Status	*Number (percentage)*
Living alone	45 (44)
Living with partner (unmarried)	21 (20)
Living with spouse	25 (24)
Living with family/friends (not partner)	12 (12)

Table 4.8   Nominal data describing marital status

Status	Number (percentage)
Living alone	38 (32)
Living with partner (unmarried)	35 (30)
Living with spouse	33 (28)
Living with family/friends (not partner)	12 (10)

A final warning

All sorts of data can be encountered. A general rule is not to push data straight into a formula. You need to think whether the formula makes sense for those data. There is always an exception to 'prove the rule'. For example, in economic analyses it is very common to obtain right-skewed data for costs. You might therefore think that the obvious summary statistic is the median. However, if the purpose of the study is to estimate the *total* cost, or to compare estimates of the total costs for two or more regimes, it is the total (or equivalently the mean) which is most appropriate.[4]

A different problem is illustrated by the data shown in Table 4.9.

Table 4.9   An example of censored data – the highest two values are not known

Value	Frequency
10	1
18	1
20	2
21	3
22	2
>24	2

Here you are given all of the data values except the largest two. All you know about the latter is that they are *at least* 24. You do not know how much greater than 24 they are. These data are *censored*. You should try to avoid obtaining data like these if possible, but sometimes it is impossible to avoid them. Such data commonly occur if you are studying *times to events of interest* (e.g. times to death, times to recurrence of a disease, times to full recovery). If some individuals take a long time to reach the event of interest, then your study might not be long enough to observe the event. In some cases, such as cases of recurrence of a disease, the recurrence might *never* be observed. Data like these are called *survival data*, and special methods are used to analyse them. What you must *not* do is calculate summary statistics omitting the censored values. Doing this for the data shown in Table 4.9 would underestimate both the mean and the standard deviation. Worse still, you might be omitting the very data that were of most interest in the study. In this case you could quote the median and interquartile range, since these are not affected by the two highest values. The median would be 21 and the interquartile range would be 20 to 22 units.

However, censored values are not always the largest values. Some people may drop out of your study (especially if it lasts a long time) or move out of the area. This could result in data like those shown in Table 4.10.

Table 4.10 An example of censored data; values marked with an asterisk are known to be at least that high, but the actual value is not known

Value	Frequency
10	1
18	1*
20	1,1*
21	3
22	1,1*
>24	2*

Here an asterisk indicates a censored value. Therefore there is one person with the time recorded as 10 units, 1 with *at least* 18 units, one with 20 units, one with *at least* 20 units, and so on. For these data, the median and quartiles cannot be calculated directly. All of the data are informative, so the analysis should include all values, but none of the plots from Chapter 3 or the summary statistics from this chapter can be used. In this case it is impossible to compute the median directly from the data, as you cannot order the data values. Special data require special methods. There are many different statistical methods available for data summary and analysis.[5,6]

Censored data are a type of missing data. Great care must be taken when handling missing values in data. You cannot just analyse the complete data and pretend that no data are missing.

When subjects do drop out from studies, you need to know what to do with their data. For randomised controlled trials it is considered good practice to analyse the data using an *intention-to-treat analysis*. This means that you include for each group the data from all of the patients who were randomised to that group. This means including dropouts and patients who even changed treatment during the study. There are very good reasons for doing this, and it is commonly accepted in principle. However, there is little consensus about how it should be done in practice.[7]

Summary

Summary statistics are numerical values that describe the key features of data.

- It is important to describe the spread as well as average values.
- The summary statistics you can use depend on the type of data and what you are trying to show.
- The mean and standard deviation are useful for symmetrical continuous data.
- The median and range or interquartile range are useful for most asymmetrical continuous data and ordinal data.
- For nominal data you should use counts and percentages or the mode.
- Counts can be misleading without percentages, and vice versa – they should be quoted together.
- Boxplots show minimum and maximum values, quartiles and the median. They are useful for investigating symmetry/skewness.
- Learn to look critically at summary statistics – do not assume that appropriate ones have been used.

CHAPTER FIVE

What's so normal about normality?

Chapter 4 discussed symmetrical and skewed data. A symmetrical histogram could have many shapes, but there is one shape of particular interest – the normal distribution. Many statistical theories and methods are intended for normally distributed data. This chapter will therefore explore several of the key features of normal distributions. Some of the material is somewhat technical, but the results are very important.

After reading this chapter you should be able to:

- recognise the shape of normally distributed data
- distinguish between a sample mean and a population mean
- understand the key role of the standard deviation for normal data
- understand why normal distribution results are applicable to a wide range of data.

The general shape of normally distributed data

Normal data are symmetrical and *bell-shaped*. Figure 5.1 illustrates the shape of three sets of normally distributed data. Histograms of the *whole population* would have these forms. All three curves have the same basic shape, but two of them are flatter, more squashed bell-shapes than the other one. For two of the curves the mean is 20 units. You can see that although one of these curves is peaked and the other one is flatter, they are both centred on their mean value of 20 units. The other curve is centred on its mean value of 25 units. Its shape is identical to the curves for a mean of 20 and a standard deviation of 3, but it is shifted along so that it is centred on 25. The more peaked curve is centred on 20 units, but it is more concentrated around this value. It has less variability – that is, less spread. It should come as little surprise, therefore, to learn that its standard deviation is lower. In fact, the standard deviation is one unit. A normal distribution is defined by its mean and standard deviation. The mean can be any value (negative, zero or positive), and the standard deviation can be any positive value. Consequently, there are very many normal distributions, but they all share the same properties, which will be discussed in this chapter. The mean defines the centre of the distribution. For a normal distribution, the mean and median are both equal to this central value. The standard deviation describes the spread of the distribution. Distributions with high standard deviations are flatter, whereas those with low standard deviations are peaked and concentrated around the central value. They all appear bell-shaped.

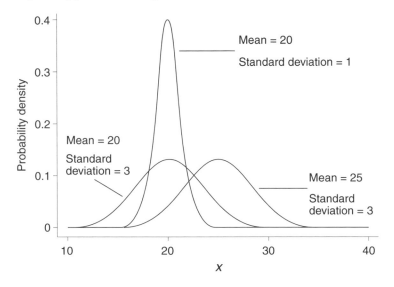

Figure 5.1 Shapes of three normal distributions. Each is defined by its mean and standard deviation.

Knowing the shape is like having data from the whole population. Statistically you would say that you knew the *distribution* of the data. The distribution is the shape of the histogram for the entire population. The mean and standard deviation are *parameters* of the distribution. In practice, it is extremely rare to have all of this information. Usually you take a sample from the population and investigate its properties. The mean and standard deviation that you then calculate depend on the particular sample that you are using – both values are subject to *variability*. A different sample will give different values. In contrast, the values of the parameters never change. Parameters are denoted by Greek letters. For the normal distribution the mean is denoted by μ and the standard deviation is denoted by σ. The *sample* mean and standard deviation are denoted by the English letters $\bar{x}$ and s.

In order to illustrate how the sample mean and standard deviation vary from one sample to another, several samples were drawn from the normal

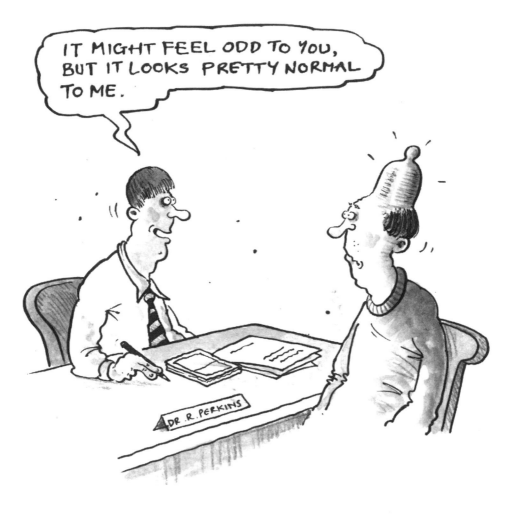

What's so normal about normality?

distribution with a mean value of 20 and a standard deviation of two. Five samples of sizes 10, 20 and 100 were drawn. Figures 5.2 to 5.4 show boxplots of the data.

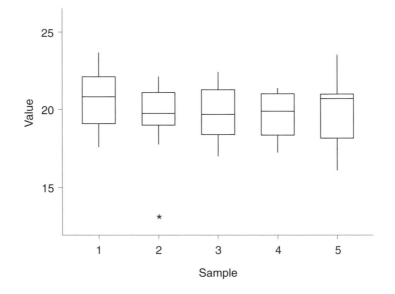

Figure 5.2 Boxplots of five samples of size 10 from a normal distribution with mean of 20 and standard deviation of two. Because the samples are so small, the quartiles and boxplots do not tell us much.

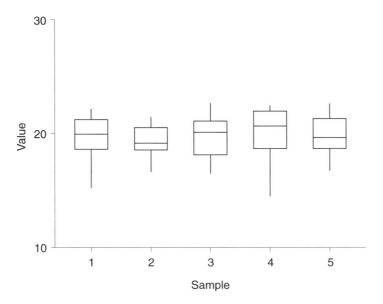

Figure 5.3 Boxplots of five samples of size 20 from a normal distribution with a mean of 20 and a standard deviation of two.

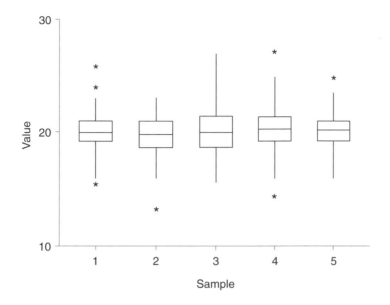

Figure 5.4 Boxplots of five samples of size 100 from a normal distribution with a mean of 20 and a standard deviation of two.

A sample of size 10 is small, and you cannot expect to draw strong conclusions from such a sample. The quartiles and boxplots cannot be very informative – the values and shapes could change quite dramatically if one of the data values changed slightly. None the less, sample 2 from the samples of size 10 (shown in Figure 5.2) has an outlier which is a long way from the rest of the data, while sample 5 looks very skewed. Figure 5.5 shows the histogram for sample 2. This appears to be negatively skewed, but remember that the sample is small. A sample of size 20 is of moderate size, and such samples are shown in Figure 5.3. The apparent skewness is less marked, and there are no outliers. The boxplots more closely resemble what we might expect for normal data. Figure 5.4 shows the boxplots for samples of size 100. These are large samples. The box parts of the plots look quite similar (remember to look at the vertical scales). There are several outliers, but there are few in relation to the 100 values in each sample. It is quite usual to obtain an odd high or low value by chance in a large sample. Figure 5.6 shows a histogram of sample 2 from Figure 5.4. With the exception of the low outlier value, the histogram looks fairly symmetrical and bell-shaped. When the sample size is as large as 500, the distribution of the data really starts to resemble the shape of Figure 5.1. Figure 5.7 shows a histogram for a sample of 500 from this normal distribution.

Table 5.1 gives the sample mean and standard deviation for each of the samples shown in the boxplots. The means are all about 20 and the standard deviations about two, but the values do vary from one sample to another. You

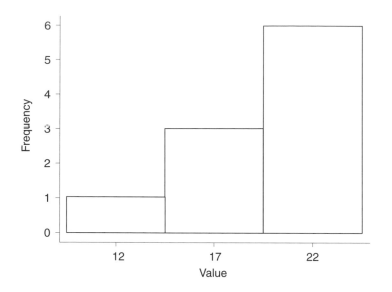

Figure 5.5   Histogram of sample 2 from Figure 5.2.

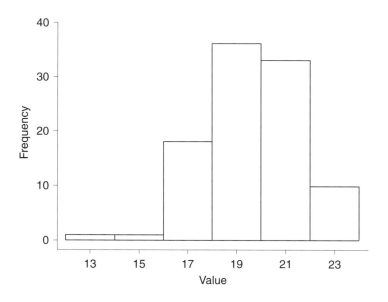

Figure 5.6   Histogram of sample 2 from Figure 5.4.

would generally have more confidence in an estimate from a larger sample than in one from a small sample. Of course, by chance you could obtain good estimates from a small sample, but in practice you would not know that you had 'struck lucky'.

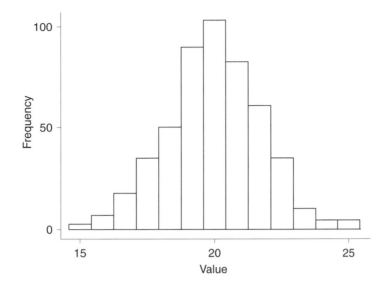

Figure 5.7   Histogram of sample of size 500 from a normal distribution with a mean of 20 and a standard deviation of two.

Table 5.1   Summary statistics for the samples from a normal distribution with a mean of 20 and a standard deviation of two

Sample	Mean	Standard deviation
$n = 10$		
1	20.8	2.0
2	19.5	2.6
3	19.9	1.9
4	19.8	1.6
5	20.0	2.4
$n = 20$		
1	19.9	1.8
2	19.5	1.3
3	19.7	1.8
4	20.2	2.4
5	19.9	2.2
$n = 100$		
1	20.0	1.9
2	19.5	1.9
3	19.7	2.3
4	20.2	2.2
5	19.9	1.8

Some normal distributions are more peaked than others, but all of them have the same basic shape. The rule of thumb given in Chapter 4 relates specifically to normal distributions. It is repeated here:

- 68% of values lie within one standard deviation of the mean
- 95% of values lie within two standard deviations of the mean
- over 99% of values lie within three standard deviations of the mean.

This rule applies irrespective of the population mean and standard deviation, and can be very useful. If you know the mean and standard deviation of a normal distribution you will have a fairly good idea of the distribution of values you are likely to obtain. This can be of great practical use, as is shown in the following example.

Study of obesity in childhood (Case Study B)

It is known that there are associations between low birth weight and increased risk of disease in adulthood. In many cases this is linked with obesity. Some infants who are small or thin at birth exhibit 'catch-up' growth in the first two years of life. This may be associated with later obesity and hence increased risk of disease. In a study which started in 1991, researchers monitored the weights of 848 infants who were full-term singletons.[1] Weights were measured at birth, then every 4 months to 12 months, then every 6 months to 4 years, and at 5 years.

The researchers used the UK growth reference data for 1990 as *population* data. At each time when an infant in the study was weighed, the population mean and standard deviation were read off the 1990 data, taking into account age and gender. A new score, called a standard deviation score (SD score), was then created:

$$\text{SD score} = \frac{(\text{actual weight} - \text{population weight})}{\text{population standard deviation}}.$$

A negative score denoted a baby who was underweight relative to the population, and a positive score denoted a baby who was overweight relative to the population. The size of the score described, in terms of standard deviations, how under- or overweight the infant was. Measuring differences in terms of standard deviations is useful because of what is known about normal distributions and standard deviations.

In fact, standard growth charts are marked in bands of 0.67 standard deviations. A change of 0.67 standard deviations moves from the second to the ninth percentile, from the ninth to the 25th percentile, and from the 25th to the 50th percentile. This is illustrated in Figure 5.8.

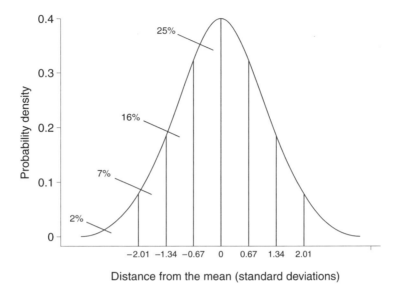

Figure 5.8 Graph of a normal distribution, showing the bands defined by intervals of 0.67 standard deviations from the mean. The percentages are the percentages of values expected in each region.

The percentages marked are the percentages of infants expected to fall within that band of weights on the graph. Thus 50% are expected to lie within 0.67 standard deviations of the mean. For normal data the quartiles are 0.67 standard deviations away from the mean (which is also the median). Only about 4% lie more than two standard deviations away from the mean – 2% in each tail. Facts like this are used to construct the growth charts that are commonly used in healthcare. Such examples show that you can measure changes such as growth in terms of standard deviations, as opposed to centimetres. Measures in standard deviations are useful if you want to make a comparison with a 'norm' or usual values.

In this study the researchers used this information in the following way:

> Changes in SD scores between birth and 2 years were calculated for weight and length (scores at 2 years minus scores at birth) and were adjusted for gestational age. A gain in SD score for weight between 0 and 2 years that was greater than 0.67 SD scores was taken to indicate clinically significant catch-up growth …. Similarly, a decrease in SD scores for weight by more than 0.67 SD scores indicated catch-down growth.

Methods similar to this are used in other areas of health (e.g. to compare bone density with population data when screening for osteoporosis).

Transformations

The authors treated the weight data as if they were normally distributed. This was not true of the other variables that they measured.

In this paper the authors report the following:

Natural logarithms of percentage body fat, total fat mass and waist circumference were calculated, as these were then normally distributed; geometric means ... are therefore presented for these variables.

This refers to a technique that is sometimes used to handle non-normal data, so you might need to know about it. If you find the following section difficult, it can be omitted.

The variables 'percentage body fat', 'total fat mass' and 'circumference' were right-skewed. This is not uncommon for biological data. Other variables such as 'time to an event' and 'age at onset of a disease' are often right-skewed. In fact, it is relatively uncommon for biological variables to be normally distributed. The technique used by the authors was to take the natural logarithms of the values:

$$\text{new value} = \log(\text{old value}).$$

If the original data are right-skewed, then often (but not always) new data are normally distributed. This is evidently what the researchers found in this study. As an illustration, consider the right-skewed data shown in Figure 4.4. The histogram is repeated here as Figure 5.9. The shape for this distribution is shown in Figure 5.10. Figure 5.11 shows the histogram of the new log values, formed in the manner described above.

The data in Figure 5.11 now have the characteristic bell-shape. This is an instance of a situation where this 'trick' has worked. Formally the method is referred to as a *transformation*. The transformation described here is a logarithmic transformation. Although the method is useful, it does not work for all right-skewed data. There are other transformations, but they are not widely used in medical research. One reason is that the summary statistics for the transformed data are not always easy to interpret. This is why the authors refer to the 'geometric mean'. Basically the mean of the transformed data is a mean of logs of the original values. *This is not the same as the log of the mean of the original data.*

In order to illustrate this, consider a data set of just two values, 1.5 and 3.7.

The mean of the original data is therefore (1.5 + 3.7)/2 = 2.6.

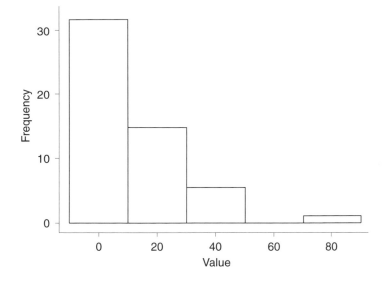

Figure 5.9   Histogram of right-skewed data (as in Figure 4.4).

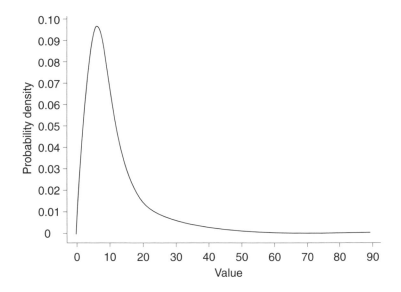

Figure 5.10   Shape of the distribution of the data shown in Figure 5.9.

And
log(1.5) = 0.405
log(3.7) = 1.308.
So the mean of the transformed data is (0.405 + 1.308)/2 = 0.857.
But the log of the mean of the original data is log(2.6) = 0.956.
In fact, 0.857 is the log of √(1.5 × 3.7).

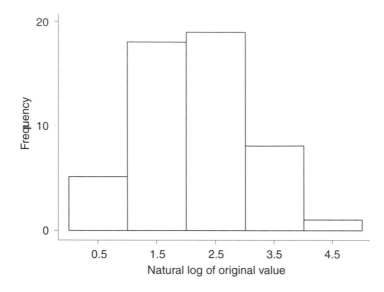

Figure 5.11 Histogram of the logs of the values shown in Figure 5.9. The transformed data appear to be normally distributed.

This expression with the square root is termed the *geometric mean* of two values. (It gets more complicated for more than two values, and you will be spared the details here.) Suffice it to say that the geometric mean is similar to the median, but lower than the ordinary mean (which is strictly called the *arithmetic mean*). Results about the mean of the transformed data can therefore be converted back into statements about the geometric mean of the original data. There is no such conversion for the standard deviation of the transformed data. Interpreting summary statistics from other types of transformation is even more difficult. Transformations can be very useful, but must be approached with care. Many people are very sceptical about the process of transforming data, believing it to be a rather dishonest trick used by statisticians who are determined to force the data into the shape that they want. There can be good reasons for using a logarithmic transformation, but these should be stated, and the results should always be presented in terms of the original scale on which the data were measured.

If so few biological data are normally distributed, and transformations are not a panacea for all problems of skewness, you might well ask what all the fuss is about with regard to this 'normal' distribution. After all, it appears to be fairly 'abnormal'. Well, the reason is embodied in a very important theorem called the *central limit theorem*.

All roads lead to Rome ...

When you take a sample and compute the sample mean, it is more often the *population* mean in which you are really interested. You use the sample mean to *estimate* the population mean. Similarly, if you are comparing the effects of two drugs, and you design a study in which one sample of patients takes one drug and a second sample takes the other drug, it is not the average effects on those particular patients that you are really interested in. You are usually interested in the mean effects among patients in general (i.e. the populations of which the samples are representative). If you are using the sample mean to estimate the population mean, you need to have some idea of how good an estimate it is. The sample mean is a statistic, not a parameter. Its value will depend on the particular sample that you used. But how does its value vary from one random sample to another? How likely are you to obtain a sample mean that is a long way away from the population mean? Are you more likely to underestimate the population mean or to overestimate it? In asking these questions you are asking about the *distribution* of the sample mean. Since in practice you will only have one value, you cannot explore this distribution using a histogram or a chart.

The central limit theorem gives you powerful results about the distribution of the sample mean. The theorem basically states that (with a few rather bizarre exceptions) whatever the shape of the original distribution, the distribution of the sample mean is approximately normal, provided that the sample is large enough.

This all sounds rather vague. You might ask how big 'large enough' would be. This is a good question, and the annoying answer is that it depends on the actual original distribution. You might also ask what is meant by 'approximately normal'. For distributions that are mildly skewed, samples of about 30 are generally regarded as 'safe'. For wildly asymmetrical distributions, the samples may have to be as large as 100. A powerful feature of the theorem is that you can estimate the mean and standard deviation of this normal distribution from the original data.

This is all best illustrated with an example.

Consider again the skewed data shown in Figure 5.10. The histogram in Figure 5.9 shows data from *one* sample of size 50. A computer can take a large number of random samples from a particular distribution. Figure 5.12 shows a histogram of 500 values. Each of these values is the sample mean from a sample of size 20 from this distribution. In other words, 500 samples each of size 20 were taken from this distribution. For each of the 500 samples, a single value – the sample mean – was extracted. These 500 values form the data for the histogram, which gives a fairly good idea of the distribution of sample means of size 20 for this distribution. It is right-skewed. Figure 5.13 is again based on 500 values, but this time the means are from samples of size 30. The skewness is still evident. However, the data shown in Figure 5.14, which is based on samples of size 100, now appear normal. This was a highly skewed initial distribution; the sample means look approximately normal for samples of size 100.

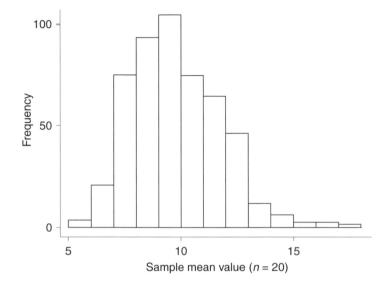

Figure 5.12   Histogram of sample means from 500 samples of size 20 from the highly right-skewed distribution shown in Figure 5.10.

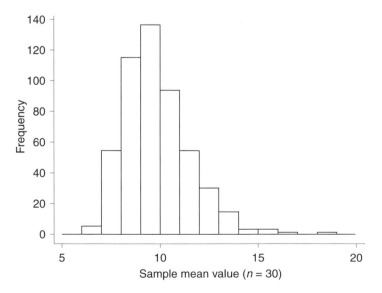

Figure 5.13   Histogram of sample means from 500 samples of size 30 from the highly right-skewed distribution shown in Figure 5.10.

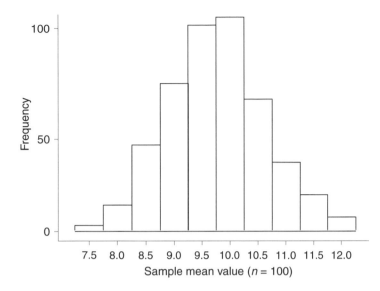

Figure 5.14 Histogram of sample means from 500 samples of size 100 from the highly right-skewed distribution shown in Figure 5.10. This appears bell-shaped.

The data shown in Figure 4.3 were right-skewed, but not as much as those in Figure 4.4. The shape for the data in Figure 4.3 is shown in Figure 5.15. It is moderately right-skewed. Based on the rules of thumb given above, you might expect that a sample of size 30 might be 'large enough' for the theorem to hold. Figure 5.16, which shows a histogram of 500 sample means from

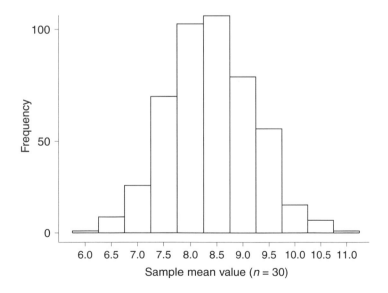

Figure 5.15 Shape of a slightly right-skewed distribution.

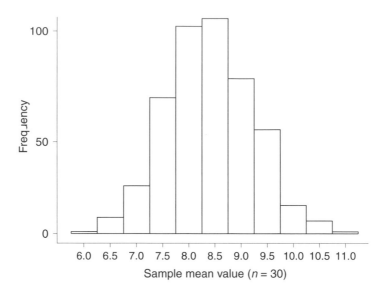

Figure 5.16   Histogram of sample means from 500 samples of size 30 from the slightly right-skewed distribution shown in Figure 5.15. It appears bell-shaped.

samples of size 30 for this distribution, confirms this to be the case. The histogram does indeed appear bell-shaped.

Here, then, is the power of this theorem. Suppose that you are doing some research to find out about a population mean. Even if your data are slightly skewed, if you have a large sample you will be able to apply the very powerful properties of the normal distribution to the sample mean.

Warning

The central limit theorem does nothing to conquer the problems of censored or missing data. These still require special treatment.

Throughout this chapter the term 'sample' has been used to denote a *random sample*. The results will not hold if you select *special* types of data from a population. Such a sample would not be representative of the population.

Summary

Normally distributed data are bell-shaped. There are many normal distributions, and each is defined by its mean and standard deviation.

• Many statistical methods are intended for normal data.

- The mean and standard deviation of a distribution are generally not known, and are often estimated from a sample.
- Small samples from a normal distribution may not look 'normal'.
- Few biological data are normally distributed.
- Taking logs of right-skewed data might result in transformed data that are approximately normal.
- The sample mean of a 'large' random sample will be approximately normally distributed.

CHAPTER SIX

Hypothesis not hype

If you take a sample of patients and measure some characteristic, it is possible (but not very likely) that your research question applies exclusively to that sample. More generally you hope that the sample is representative of some much larger *population*. You therefore use the information in the sample to make inferences about the population. This involves the use of confidence intervals and statistical tests.

After reading this chapter you should be able to:

*   interpret confidence intervals
*   distinguish between standard error and standard deviation
*   describe the principles of statistical tests
*   interpret *P*-values
*   appreciate why confidence intervals are more informative than *P*-values.

Confidence intervals

When you calculate summary statistics such as the mean and standard deviation, your calculation is from the sample data (since that is all that you have), but you are probably really interested in the mean and standard deviation of the population. Your sample values are *estimates* of the values for the population, whereas the population values are known as *parameters*. The values of parameters are seldom known. If, by chance, you had chosen a different sample, the population parameters would be just the same, but your sample estimates would be slightly different. The estimates depend on the sample taken. This is because of natural variability. As was discussed in Chapter 4, this variability between samples will be less if your samples are larger, as larger samples give more precise estimates. In small samples you are likely to get odd extreme values which can have an influence on the estimates, but this influence is much less in larger samples. It follows that your *confidence* in the estimates depends on the *size* of the sample you took. Clearly it will also depend on the *variability* in the population from which you are sampling.

Ideally, then, you want to obtain some idea of the uncertainty associated with your estimates. The variability associated with the original variable – the population – is called the *population standard deviation*. The variability of an estimate is called a *standard error*.

Recall that for the normal distribution it is possible to make statements such as the following:

*   95% of values lie within two standard deviations of the mean
*   over 99% of values lie within three standard deviations of the mean.

A similar idea is used to produce *confidence intervals* for a parameter. Here are some examples:

*   a 95% confidence interval for the population mean is 18.3 to 21.3 units
*   a 99% confidence interval for the population mean is 17.8 to 21.8 units.

These examples are taken from the sample shown in Figure 4.2. In this case, because the data were simulated, the population mean is actually *known* to be 20 units. The sample mean was 19.8, the standard deviation was 5.3 and the standard error of the mean was 0.75 units. The confidence intervals are interpreted as follows. In the first case, we are 95% sure that the range of values between 18.3 and 21.3 units contains the true population mean. In the second case, the confidence is higher at 99%, so the confidence interval needs to be wider. Note that you cannot be sure that you have caught the true value, although in this case both confidence intervals do actually contain the population mean.

In practice this means that if you took 100 *independent* (unrelated) random samples from the same population, and for each one you calculated a 95% confidence interval for the population mean, about 95 of the 100 samples would actually contain the mean, and the other five would not. Unfortunately, in practice you would have only one sample, and you could not be sure whether you had one of the 95 or one of the five.

Consider the following example. Figures 6.1 to 6.3 show the results of a simulation. In each case 100 samples have been drawn from a normal distribution with a mean of 20. For each sample a 95% confidence interval has been calculated, and these have then been ordered to make a 'pretty' graph. Each horizontal line shows a confidence interval. The vertical line shows the actual population mean. Figure 6.1 shows data from samples of size 20 where the standard deviation is two. In Figure 6.2 the standard deviation is still two, but the samples are of size 50. In Figure 6.3 the samples are of size 50, but the standard deviation is five.

Within each figure the confidence intervals vary in both location and width. This is due to chance in the sampling. In Figure 6.1, two intervals are too low to catch the true value of 20, and two intervals are too high. In Figure 6.2, three intervals are low and four are high, but overall the

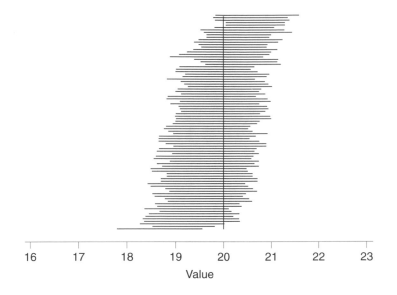

Figure 6.1   One hundred confidence intervals from samples of size 20 from a normal distribution with a mean of 20 and a standard deviation of two. Of these, 96/100 contain the true value of 20.

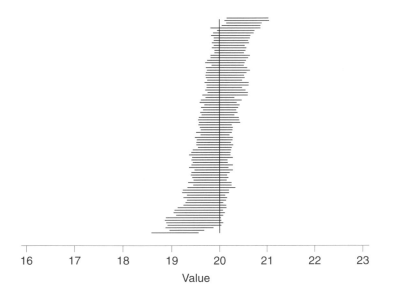

Figure 6.2   One hundred confidence intervals from samples of size 50 from a normal distribution with a mean of 20 and a standard deviation of two. Of these, 93/100 contain the true value of 20.

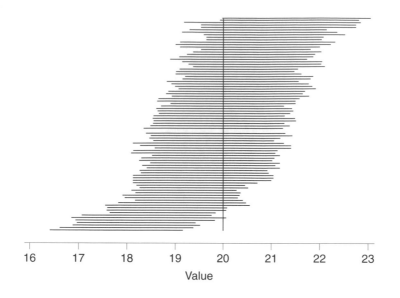

Figure 6.3   One hundred confidence intervals from samples of size 50 from a normal distribution with a mean of 20 and a standard deviation of five. Of these, 93/100 contain the true value of 20.

confidence intervals are narrower than in Figure 6.1, because they are based on larger samples. In contrast, the confidence intervals in Figure 6.3 are wider than those in Figure 6.2, because although the samples are of size 50, the population standard deviation is greater, at a value of five. For Figure 6.3, seven confidence intervals are low, and none are too high. Overall, in each figure about 95 out of 100 confidence intervals contain the actual mean, as we expected.

In practice, given a sample we can be reasonably sure that a confidence interval, if correctly computed, contains the population mean. The best estimate of the population mean is the sample mean, but as is clear from the figures it may be that the population mean is really near the end of a confidence interval. The end-values of a confidence interval may be values which are clinically very significant and which would warrant further investigation. Confidence intervals are therefore very informative.

Instead of giving a confidence interval, some researchers quote the *standard error* of a parameter estimate. A standard error has the same role as a standard deviation. The standard error of an estimate of the population mean is called the standard error of the mean. Just as the standard deviation gives a measure of the variability in the population, the standard error of the mean gives a measure of the variability of the estimate of the mean. The standard error of the mean is *less than* the population standard deviation. Careless researchers sometimes mix standard errors and standard deviations, giving a very confused picture as a result. Make sure that you know the difference between the two, and which is being quoted. Standard deviations are summary statistics, whereas standard errors are statistics used for making inferences.

Confidence intervals and standard errors do not just apply to estimates of the population mean. They can and should be calculated for any estimates of population parameters that are based on samples. The method used to compute an estimate will usually employ information about the distribution of the original population. If wrong assumptions are made, the confidence interval or standard error may not be valid. It is therefore very important to know as much as possible about the distribution of the data. This involves the results of previous research, clinical knowledge and common sense.

The basic ideas are best illustrated by examples.

Examples of confidence intervals

In the study of the nurse consultation system,[1] one of the adverse events that was counted was the number of deaths over the study period within seven days of the telephone call when the nurse consultation system was in place. The number quoted is 58, with a 95% confidence interval of 44 to 75. The best estimate based on the study data is 58 deaths. However, the study was conducted on a sample of patients over a particular period of time. The aim of the study was to estimate what would be likely to happen in general, subject to the same conditions. It is the population of all such study periods, not just this sample, that is therefore of principal interest. The population value could reasonably be as high as 75 or as low as 44. The higher limit must be the one of prime interest, since the count is of adverse effects.

The study also reported the number of hospital admissions within 24 hours of a call when the nurse consultation system was in place. This value is given as 375, with a 95% confidence interval of 339 to 414 admissions. Note again how the confidence interval gives much more information than the point estimate, and it is the higher limit that is of greatest clinical interest.

In the study of the effects of the television drama on overdoses,[2] the main objective was to investigate the influence of the *Casualty* programme, so it was necessary to compare the numbers of overdoses before and after the broadcast. The paper quotes percentage changes, 95% confidence intervals and *P*-values for presentation rates over the two 3-week periods. Examples are given below.

- For all overdoses the percentage change is 7%, with a 95% confidence interval of 0% to 15%, and $P = 0.05$.

- For females the percentage change is 13%, with a 95% confidence interval of 5% to 21%, and $P = 0.001$.
- For non-paracetamol overdoses the percentage change is 2%, with a 95% confidence interval of -7% to 12%, and $P = 0.6$.

If you have read any paper that included statistics, it is likely to have been peppered with such *P-values*. These are related to *hypothesis tests*.

Hypothesis tests

Before we look at hypothesis tests, consider the confidence intervals given in the previous section. First note that the researchers have chosen to look at the *percentage* change in presentation rates, not just differences. Why is this? When reading a report like this you should check that the statistics which are presented make sense. Here the presentation rate before the broadcast varied from one hospital to another. So an increase of two on an initial rate of five is more impressive than the same increase of two but on an initial rate of seven. You might reasonably expect a greater increase where the initial rate was higher. A percentage change reflects this, so a sensible statistic has in fact been used.

The researchers were looking for possible effects of the programme. If the programme had no effect, then the percentage changes in the population would be zero. The values in the sample might not be exactly zero – they might be positive or negative, but these non-zero values would just be chance occurrences. For the non-paracetamol overdoses the estimated percentage change is positive at a value of 2%. However, the confidence interval ranges from a *decrease* of 7% to an *increase* of 12%. The evidence for a programme effect on non-paracetamol overdoses seems to be weak.

In contrast, the presentation rate for females increases by 13% with a confidence interval of 5% to 21%. Even the lowest value of the confidence interval is an increase of 5%. Here there seems to be strong evidence that the programme has an effect, and that it is a deleterious one.

For overall overdoses the situation is less clear. The estimate is an increase of 7%, but the confidence interval ranges from 0% (no effect) to 15%. It seems as if, on balance, the programme has had a deleterious effect, but the effect could be zero or negligible.

In this example the statistic of interest is the percentage change in presentation rates. The value for 'no effect' is 0%. A confidence interval which contains zero is consistent with no overall effect, whereas a confidence interval which lies entirely on one side of 0% suggests that the programme did have an effect. The evidence for an effect is stronger when the confidence interval is further away from 0%.

In this study the researchers were trying to show that the programme did have an effect (and in fact to quantify that effect). The research question is therefore 'Is there a change in the weekly rate of presentations after the broadcast compared with that before it?'. (You might think that they should be looking for an increase. However, it is conceivable that people could be deterred from making suicide attempts. The programme did highlight the dangers of liver poisoning, and one patient said 'I didn't want to wake up with liver damage and have a slow death'. Unless it is impossible, or of no practical interest, to look for a change in one direction, you should always look for a change.) To perform a statistical test you need the following:

1   a test statistic
2   a pair of hypotheses:
    •   a null hypothesis
    •   an alternative hypothesis.

The null hypothesis defines 'no effect'. Here the following statements hold.

•   The test statistic is the percentage change in weekly presentation rate.
•   The null hypothesis is that the percentage change is zero.
•   The alternative hypothesis is that the percentage change is not zero.

Remember that it is the population value that is of interest, not the sample value. The hypotheses are referring to the population parameter, and the test statistic is based on the sample.

In a different situation you might be looking for a change, as opposed to a percentage change. Then the following statements would hold.

•   The test statistic could be an average (sample) difference.
•   The null hypothesis could be that the average (population) difference is zero.
•   The alternative hypothesis could be that the average (population) difference is not zero.

If you were interested in ratios:

•   the test statistic could be a (sample) ratio
•   the null hypothesis could be that the (population) ratio is 1
•   the alternative hypothesis could be that the (population) ratio is not 1.

The test statistic is therefore the evidence that you are going to use to decide between the two hypotheses. The procedure for this is counter-intuitive to many people. The hypotheses do not have equal status. In the absence of strong evidence against it, you choose the null hypothesis. Only if there is strong evidence against the null hypothesis do you reject it in favour of the alternative. This means that the observed value of the test statistic is unlikely to have occurred by chance if the null hypothesis is true, so there is evidence that there is something other than just chance influencing its value. Hence the following statements hold.

- A large percentage change (increase or decrease) would lead you to reject the null hypothesis of no percentage change.
- A large difference (positive or negative) would lead you to reject the null hypothesis of no difference.
- A ratio much greater or smaller than 1 would lead you to reject the null hypothesis that the ratio is 1.

At this stage you might ask, 'How large is large?'. That is a very good question. The answer is complicated. Essentially 'large' means large relative to what you would expect if the null hypothesis was true. This will depend on the actual distribution, the population standard deviation and the sample size used. And, as before, if you make false assumptions about the distribution you can obtain false results. A further complication is that statisticians do not talk about 'accepting' the null hypothesis. They either 'reject' or 'fail to reject' it. This terminology may seem perverse, but there is a good reason for it. If you do not have enough evidence to reject the null hypothesis, it could be for one of the following reasons.

- The population value is really exactly zero (or the appropriate 'no effect' value). In fact, this is fairly unlikely.
- The population value is not exactly zero, but is so small that it is of little practical interest.
- The population value is not zero, and is of real practical interest, but you failed to detect this, either because your sample was too small, or just because of bad luck.

The *P*-value is the probability of observing a test statistic at least that far away from the 'no effect' value if the null hypothesis is true. It is the probability that the apparent effect is attributable to chance when the null hypothesis is true.

Hence:

- if a *P*-value is very high there is not much evidence against the null hypothesis
- if a *P*-value is very low there is strong evidence against the null hypothesis.

Conventionally, the cut-off value is taken to be 5% or one in 20. Therefore, as a general rule, if the *P*-value is less than 0.05 you reject the null hypothesis.

In the examples from the study of overdoses it is possible to draw the following conclusions.

- For the non-paracetamol overdoses, the *P*-value is 0.6. This is very high, and therefore you would not reject the null hypothesis of no percentage increase. There is insufficient evidence that the programme influenced non-paracetamol presentation rates.

- For the paracetamol overdoses among females, the *P*-value is 0.001, which is very low, so there is strong evidence against the null hypothesis. You would conclude that for females there is evidence that the programme did cause a change in presentation rates, and that it was an increase.
- For all overdoses, the *P*-value is 0.05, which is marginal. There is evidence that suggests a deleterious effect.

Table 6.1 summarises the evidence about programme effects discussed in this section.

Table 6.1   Summary of evidence for effects of the television programme on different presentation rates

	Point estimate of percentage change	*95% confidence interval for percentage change*	*P-value*	*Interpretation*
Presentation rates for all overdoses	7	0 to 15	0.05	Suggestive evidence of a deleterious effect (confidence interval borders on zero; $P = 0.05$)
Presentation rates for females	13	5 to 21	0.001	Strong evidence of a deleterious effect (confidence interval far from zero; *P*-value very small)
Presentation rates for non-paracetamol overdoses	2	–7 to 12	0.6	Insufficient evidence of an effect (confidence interval spans zero; $P > 0.05$)

You might be wrong

The philosophy behind hypothesis testing is 'Let us assume no effect and try to prove otherwise'.

The process is like that of trying an accused person in court. The comparison is as follows:

- null hypothesis – prisoner is innocent
- alternative hypothesis – prisoner is guilty
- test statistic – evidence against the prisoner.

The verdict is 'innocent' or 'guilty'. A better analogy would be a verdict of 'not proven' or 'guilty'. None the less, the two procedures have similarities. In court, two possible mistakes could be made. The jury could convict an innocent person (falsely reject the null hypothesis) or they could let the guilty go free (falsely fail to reject the null hypothesis). If you reduce the likelihood of one type of mistake, you necessarily increase the likelihood of the other. You cannot win. In criminal trials in the UK a person is assumed to be innocent until proven guilty – the null hypothesis is not rejected unless there is a weight of evidence against it. In statistics the two types of mistake have named probabilities associated with them.

- A type I error is the probability of rejecting the null hypothesis when it is true. You do this by attributing a real effect to chance. This probability is generally kept low, and is controlled by the way in which you interpret the *P*-value. The conventional value is 5% (as above), but if you want to be strict you can use the value 1%, and if you want to be lax you can use the value 10%.
- A type II error is the probability of failing to reject the null hypothesis when it is false. This depends on both the size of the actual effect and the size of the sample taken.

It is therefore important that your study sample is large enough to have a good chance of detecting any effect or difference that is of real clinical/practical relevance. This needs to be addressed at the design stage. Failure to do this might result in your missing an effect that is of major practical significance.

Power of a test

The type II error is associated with the *power* of a test – that is, the probability that it will detect a particular effect if it exists. High power means low type II error. In general, you increase the power of a test by taking a larger sample. However, there are different types of tests. For example, *parametric* tests are used when you can reasonably make assumptions about the distribution (e.g. that it is approximately normal). *Non-parametric* tests do not require assumptions about the distribution. In general, non-parametric tests are less powerful than parametric ones; so, given the choice, you would often choose a parametric test. However, if the assumptions are not valid, then the *P*-values and confidence intervals you obtain from such a test might be inaccurate and could be wildly so.

Significance

The test statistic and associated graphs and plots of the data *describe* the evidence against the null hypothesis. A *P*-value quantifies the *size* of that evidence. A low P-value indicates strong evidence against the null hypothesis. Such a result is described as 'statistically significant'. Traditionally, the following results have applied:

- $P < 0.05$: the result is statistically significant, marked *
- $P < 0.01$: the result is statistically highly significant, marked **
- $P < 0.001$: the result is statistically very highly significant, marked ***.

(Note that $<$ means 'less than': e.g. $2 < 3$.)

Researchers vary with regard to the way in which they quote results. Ideally they should quote the *actual P*-value. However, you still see statements such as $P < 0.01$, $P > 0.05$ or, even worse, NS (which means 'not significant'). Viewing a P-value as 'strength of evidence' means that you want to know the actual value. Furthermore, and in some ways more importantly, you want to know the potential size of an effect even if the P-value is high. For this reason, P-values without estimates of effects and associated confidence intervals are of little use. The reported result 'NS' tells you next to nothing. Even if the P-value is high, the confidence interval might contain values that are of great practical interest, and you would want to know this.

In fact, the interpretation of tests is not a simple matter of comparing a P-value with some predetermined cut-off value. This mechanistic approach is very outdated. A mechanistic rule would reject the null hypothesis if $P = 0.049$ and not reject it if $P = 0.052$, but no one in their right mind would think that there was much to choose between these two P-values, which are effectively the same. The acceptable approach is more a matter of judgement, taking into account what is already known, the P-value obtained from the test, and the confidence interval. It is much more useful to describe effects, your confidence in them, and the implications, than merely to 'hide behind' an apparently small P-value. Sadly, there needs to be something of a culture change for people to do this.

Another important point is that statistical significance does not imply practical significance. If you take a very large sample, you might find strong evidence for an effect of little practical interest. For example, suppose you were comparing two sets of sleeping tablets. You give the tablets to one set of patients and an indistinguishable placebo to another set. Assume that the study is well designed. You find very strong evidence that the tablets give, on average, 10 minutes more sleep than the placebo does. However low the P-value may be, this finding is unlikely to be of any interest.

There is an example of the 'common-sense' or judgemental approach to P-values in the study on paracetamol overdose. The paper states that '*Casualty* viewers attending after the episode were more likely to state that general television viewing influenced their choice of drug than those attending before the broadcast (14% vs. 6%, $P = 0.1$)'.[2]

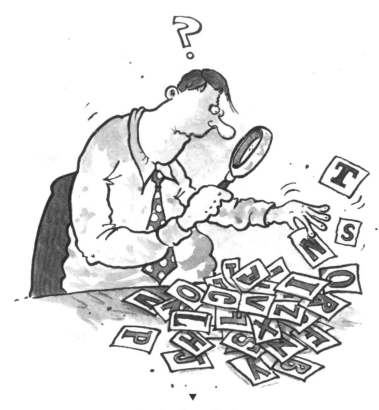

▼

Hunting for a *P*-value

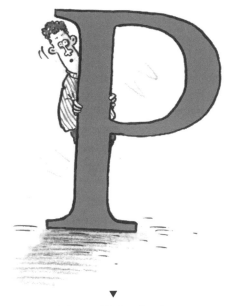

▼

Hiding behind a *P*-value

Traditionally, a P-value of 0.1 would not be regarded as low. However, the percentages quoted are based on very small subsets of the whole study sample. The value after the episode is 10/69 and that before it is 4/71. Therefore the sample sizes are small and the test will have low power. However, this observed difference is large enough to be of potential interest, and the authors are correct to report it in this way, making it clear that the evidence for it is not strong. Had this result been a primary objective of the study, the lack of power would have compromised the results. However, the study was large enough to be able to quantify the main effects.

For the main results, researchers should describe their data, state which test they are performing, and give not only P-values but also confidence intervals for all effects of interest.[3] Only then can the statistical and clinical relevance of the findings be assessed, and the results obtained from different studies be compared.

That summarises the basics of statistical tests. However, there are more ramifications, although the remainder of this chapter could be omitted from a first reading.

Comparing baseline measures

Many studies involve the comparison of two groups that have been given different treatments. You want any observed difference in outcome between the two groups to be attributable to the treatments. This means that in all other respects the two groups must be as similar as possible. A method that is often used to try to achieve this is random allocation of patients to the two groups. A set of baseline measures is then taken on the two groups, and they are compared. In the literature it is common to see a table of summary statistics comparing the baseline measures of the two groups. This is good. The table usually contains P-values for tests of no differences. This is futile.[4] If you *know* that the groups were allocated by chance, then any differences between them must be attributable to chance. There is no point in testing for something you know. It is much more profitable to examine the summary statistics. Irrespective of the P-values, there may be differences between the groups (which have occurred by chance) which might influence the results. You should watch out for this. If authors are 'hiding behind' P-values, they might miss important information. If there are apparent differences between the groups, you should question whether they might have influenced the results, even if the authors have not been wise enough to do this themselves.

The hunt for a *P*-value

Another bad practice is to test as many things as you can in the hope of eventually finding something that has a low *P*-value – 'hunt the *P*-value'. The problem with this approach is that you will end up performing a large number of tests. This is called *multiple testing*. If you perform one test, taking a significance level of 5%, then you will expect to find a spuriously 'interesting' effect about once in every 20 times you perform the test. Therefore if you carry out 20 different tests in your study, you can expect to get about one significant result by chance. For this reason you should beware of studies with multiple tests. Ideally there should be one (or a small number) of pre-specified effects of prime interest. If many tests have been performed you generally need to inter-pret *P*-values more strictly. For example, researchers may state that 'Owing to the large number of tests carried out, a significance level of 0.01 was adopted', or something similar. As a general rule of thumb you need to divide the cut-off *P*-value by the number of tests you have performed. Typically, if you have carried out 10 tests you are looking for *P*-values of less than 0.005. Beware of researchers who carry out multiple tests and who stick rigidly to a 'less than 0.05' rule.

Another mistake, which is in some respects even more serious, is to devise hypotheses after looking at the data. It is common for a very large number of measurements to be taken on a set of patients. If you search around for long enough you are almost bound to find a subset (e.g. redheads under the age of 45 years) that looks different from the rest. The *P*-value associated with a test might even be very small. However, in searching for interesting subsets you will have done the equivalent of carrying out very many tests. This is called *data dredging*, which is very bad practice, and the *P*-value is probably meaningless. At best you might have found something worthy of comment and of following up in a further study. The hypotheses that are to be tested should be specified at the design stage of a study.

Other tests

When testing for a difference without specifying the direction of that difference, you are carrying out a *two-sided test*. That is, you are interested in finding either an increase or a decrease. Occasionally you might *know* that the effect can only be in one direction. If this is genuinely the case, then you carry out a *one-sided test*. This *must* be specified before data collection, because your reason for doing a one-sided test is in no way influenced by the data. If researchers have carried out one-sided tests, it should be clear that they had decided to do this during the design stage. If they have not made this clear, you should view their results with some caution, especially if the *P*-values are marginal.

In general, a result which is significant in a two-sided test will also be significant in the appropriate one-sided test, but the converse is not true. If in doubt, do a two-sided test. You need very good reasons to carry out a one-sided test.

In the examples given so far, the research question was related to 'an effect', which was reflected in the alternative hypothesis. Sometimes the research question is not matched to the alternative hypothesis. For example, if you wanted to investigate whether data were compatible with a normal distribution, you would have a pair of hypotheses:

1 null hypothesis – data are normally distributed
2 alternative hypothesis – data are not normally distributed.

The hypotheses have to be this way round because, in order to calculate a *P*-value, you need to know a lot about the distribution associated with the null hypothesis. The alternative here could be virtually any distribution. Now the default position is 'do not reject the null hypothesis', and you can easily obtain this result by simply taking a small sample. Clearly this is not what you want. As Altman says,[5] 'Absence of evidence is not evidence of absence'.

So in this case you have to try to make the power of the test high. This often means taking a more liberal view of the *P*-value, and rejecting the null hypothesis for *P*-values of up to, say, 0.1. The balance between the power and significance level of a test depends on the implications of making wrong decisions. In practice, if you have a small sample a test of normality will probably tell you very little. You will need to use clinical knowledge and common sense to judge whether or not your data are likely to be approximately normal.

A similar problem arises if you are trying to show that two treatments are equivalent. Here 'equivalent' can mean 'A is in practical terms not worse than B', or it can mean 'A is in practical terms no better and no worse than B'. In each case you are effectively trying to show 'no difference', so you must make sure that the power of the test is high, even if this means demanding a higher level of significance. In general, an equivalence test requires a larger sample than a test designed to find a difference and is constructed in a different way.[6]

All of these issues should have been discussed fully at the design stage, and should be reported in the literature. Full details must be provided, and you should be able to find them in the Methods section, possibly under a heading such as 'Design', 'Sample size' or 'Power calculation'. A paper in which this is not clear is somewhat deficient.

Summary

- Statistics based on samples are used to estimate population parameters.
- The standard error of an estimate is a measure of its precision. It is different from the standard deviation of the population.
- Confidence intervals give a range of values which you can be fairly certain contain the parameter of interest.
- *P*-values measure the strength of evidence against a null hypothesis and in favour of an alternative. They should be interpreted judgementally and not mechanistically.
- Confidence intervals should accompany *P*-values.
- Statistical significance is not the same as clinical significance.
- Studies should be designed to have sufficient power to detect clinically significant effects.
- Multiple testing and testing of hypotheses based on the data are dangerous.
- Researchers should give details of how they designed the study and planned tests to be sufficiently powerful to detect relevant effects.

CHAPTER SEVEN

Confound it

Chapter 6 contained a lot of material about *P*-values. This is because they pervade the literature. However, nowadays it is much more important to *model* data than merely to carry out statistical tests. This modelling has nothing to do with string, card or glue. It means finding equations that describe relationships between variables. This chapter is therefore about the relationships between variables.

After reading it you should be able to:

*   understand what is meant by a model
*   distinguish between association and causation
*   describe the effect of confounding and the problems it can cause
*   recognise an interaction effect.

A model?

Suppose you are studying the effect of a particular treatment. You have two groups of suitably chosen subjects. One group receives the active treatment and the other group receives a placebo. You measure some relevant characteristic before the course of treatment and then again at the end of the study. You are investigating whether or not the active treatment affects this characteristic. The initial values are called *baseline measures*. A simple way to analyse these data would be to calculate the differences by subtracting the 'after' measures from the 'before' measures, and to test the hypothesis that on average these differences are the same for each group. This is essentially the approach described in Chapter 6. However, the change in the characteristic might depend on the baseline value, as in the study on attempted suicides. You might expect a larger change when the baseline value is higher. One way of dealing with this would be to look at the percentage change in response. Another way would be to try to define a relationship between the response after treatment and the response before treatment. You would have to allow for potentially different relationships for the two groups. Moreover, if you thought that females might respond differently from males you might also want to allow for this effect. In addition, you could take measures at more than two time points, to see how the characteristic varied over time. All this together would be an example of a *model*, relating the *outcome* or *response* variable to a set of *predictor* or *explanatory* variables. The model could become extremely complicated, and you should restrict yourself to variables which you have good reason to think could influence the outcome. If you are able to do this you may be able to obtain a much more informative potential explanation of what is happening. Such a modelling procedure is not trivial. Generally, several models are investigated, as parameters are included in or excluded from the model. The ideal result is to have a model that provides an explanation for most of the features in the data, that is simple (not overly complex) and that makes clinical sense. The modeller will examine several *P*-values, and will make checks on the validity of the model during this process, which requires the following to be taken into account:

- what is already known from previous research
- the *P*-values and other information indicating how well the model describes the data
- clinical judgement
- common sense.

You may recognise that this list is similar to that given in Chapter 6 for interpreting *P*-values. The principles are similar – you do not want to include any effects that are just bizarre, 'chance' features of your sample. You want your model to be general. As with hypothesis tests, a model may be valid only if certain assumptions can be made about the data (e.g. that they are normally distributed), so these assumptions need to be checked. There are also many other checks to be made on a model. For example, it will not be a good model if the estimates of some of the parameters are overly influenced by the data from one subject. An experienced modeller will know how best to resolve these issues.

One of the simplest relationships between two variables is a straight-line relationship, and some aspects of such a model will be discussed in this chapter.

Correlation coefficient

Figure 7.1 shows two sets of artificial data, and indicates possible patterns between two variables. Because the variables are artificial, they have artificial names. The variable along the horizontal axis (traditionally called the *x*-axis) is called the *x*-variable. The variable along the vertical axis (traditionally called the *y*-axis) is called the *y*-variable. So for each set the *x*-variable takes values 1 to 10. For set 1, identified by circles, *y* increases with an increase in *x*. In fact, an increase of one unit in *x* is associated with an *increase* of three units in *y*, irrespective of the value of *x*. The points fit on a straight line with a

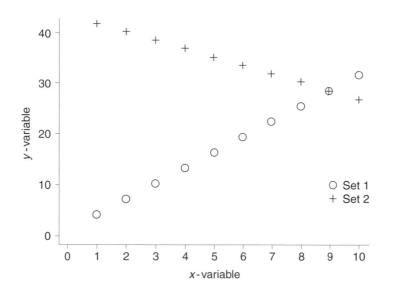

Figure 7.1 Two sets of artificial data. For set 1 there is a positive linear association, and for set 2 there is a negative linear association.

positive slope. This is described as a *positive linear association* between the two variables. The association is 'perfect'. In contrast, for set 2, denoted by plus signs, an increase of one unit in x is associated with a *decrease* of two units in y. This is a *negative linear association*. The line is less steep, but the association is still perfect.

The *correlation coefficient* is a number that measures the degree of *linear* association between two continuous variables. It takes a value between 1 and -1. The two data sets in Figure 7.1 show extreme values:

- set 1 has a correlation coefficient of $+1$: perfect positive linear association
- set 2 has a correlation coefficient of -1: perfect negative linear association.

Note that the value depends on how 'perfect' the fit to a line is, and whether the line slopes upwards (positive slope and positive value) or downwards (negative slope and negative value). It does *not* depend on the size of the slope. The slope is less steep for set 2, but the fit is still perfect.

Of course, in practice you would not see data like these. Natural variability would mean that even if a line were a good model of the association between the variables, the observed points would be scattered around a line. The plot of points is then called a scatter plot (as described in Chapter 3), and the line that is fitted using a statistical package is called the *regression line*. Figure 7.2 shows three scatter plots. Now the situation is somewhat different.

For set 1 the correlation coefficient is $+0.96$. This is a positive value close to $+1$, and reflects the fact that there is evidence of a strong positive linear

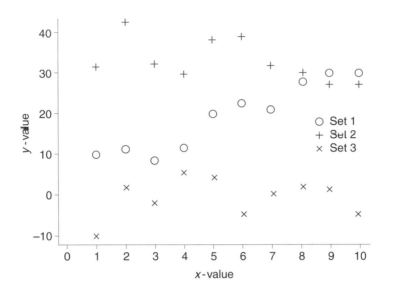

Figure 7.2   Three scatter plots of artificial data. For set 1 there is a fairly strong positive linear association, for set 2 there is a weak negative linear association, and for set 3 there is no obvious linear association.

association between the x-values and the y-values for these data. There is much more scatter in set 2. The y-value still tends to decrease with an increase in x-values, but the association is less clear. This is reflected by the value of the correlation coefficient, which is −0.61. The correlation coefficient for set 3 is +0.09, a value close to zero. For these data there is little evidence of a linear association between the two variables. Note that for all three sets any apparent fluctuations are due to chance – there is no cyclical variation in the data.

For associations between two variables, the value of the correlation coefficient *squared* means something. It describes the proportion of the variation in the y-values that can be explained by a straight-line model in the x-values. Thus in Figure 7.1, *all* of the variation in y is modelled by a straight line in x-values for sets 1 and 2. For the data in Figure 7.2 the values are as follows:

- for set 1, 92% of the variation in y can be modelled by a straight line in x
- for set 2, 37% of the variation in y can be modelled by a straight line in x
- for set 3, 0.8% of the variation in y can be modelled by a straight line in x.

A real example was given in Chapter 3, and the scatter plot of Figure 3.9 is reproduced here.

There is a weak negative association between the change in upper incisor angle and the value of the incisor angle before treatment. Note, however, that the changes are almost all negative – the angle is decreasing. Thus a lower value on the graph denotes a larger change. Remember how important it is to look at the scales. The association is not strong – there is a lot of scatter. This

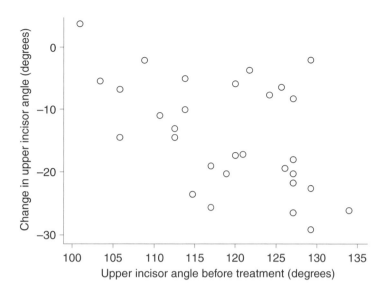

Figure 7.3   Scatter plot showing weak negative association between the change in upper incisor angle and the value of the incisor angle before treatment (as in Figure 3.9).

is reflected in a negative correlation coefficient of −0.51. This means that 26% of the variation in change in upper incisor angle is modelled by a straight-line relationship with the angle before treatment. This might be a situation in which you would look for a more complicated model. There is no evidence from the plot that the model should be a curve instead of a straight line, but there might be other *predictor* variables that can be included to improve the model. However, this book does not cover such advanced methods.

Beware of correlation coefficients

Correlation coefficients can be informative, but they must be treated with caution and also common sense. In clinical studies it is popular to measure a whole set of variables on each subject and to report correlation coefficients. The reported values are *sample statistics*, and computer packages can give you a P-value for a correlation coefficient, testing the hypothesis that the population value is really zero. For very large samples, small values of sample correlation coefficients can have very low P-values. However, low correlation coefficients are very seldom clinically significant. The correct interpretation of a correlation coefficient does not rest entirely on a P-value. In the study of postnatal catch-up growth and obesity in childhood, the authors adopted the right approach. They stated that 'The correlation between SD scores for weight at birth and at 2 years was low ($r = 0.36$, $P < 0.0005$) compared with that between 2 and

5 years ($r = 0.8$, $P < 0.0005$)'.[1] Here r denotes the sample correlation coefficient. (The population value is denoted by the Greek letter ρ.) The study had a large sample of over 800 infants. Although there is very strong evidence that the first correlation coefficient is non-zero, the authors regard its value as too low to be of clinical interest. A linear model using scores at birth only explains 13% of the variation in the scores at 2 years. In contrast, 64% of the variation in scores at 5 years is explained by a straight-line model using the scores at 2 years.

Another reason to be wary of P-values here is that if you have looked at several correlation coefficients, then you have effectively carried out several tests. The problem of multiple testing discussed in Chapter 6 rears its ugly head again.

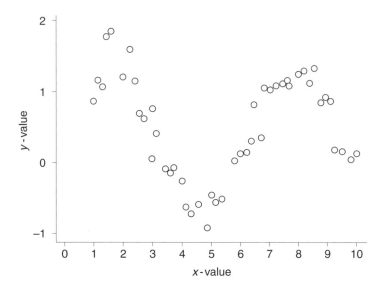

Figure 7.4   Scatter plot of data where there is a non-linear association. The correlation coefficient is low.

There are other reasons for being cautious about correlation coefficients. They only model *linear* associations. Figure 7.4 shows data where there seems to be a fairly strong non-linear association between the two variables. The correlation coefficient is −0.03, indicating little linear association. Blindly using a correlation coefficient is as pointless as blindly following or hiding behind any other statistic. It is always important to examine data using common sense.

Figure 7.5 shows a set of data where the correlation coefficient (and the straight line modelling the data) is heavily influenced by a single point. The correlation coefficient for all of the data is 0.59, which is a moderately high value. (As a rule of thumb, values greater than 0.7 or more negative than –0.7 are usually worth investigating.) However, if the point marked with a plus sign is removed, the value drops to 0.09. Any evidence of a linear association is almost entirely dominated by this outlier point. It is fairly clear from the scatter plot that the remainder of the points form a random scatter with no pattern.

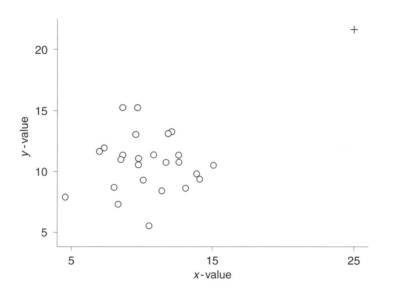

Figure 7.5 Scatter plot showing the influence of a single point on the correlation coefficient. The value is 0.59 if the + in the top right-hand corner is included, and 0.09 if it is not.

A less extreme example is given in Figure 7.6. This shows the data from Figure 7.3 with one extra point added, identified by a plus symbol. The correlation coefficient changes from –0.51 to –0.44 as a result of this extra point. Another problem with the correlation coefficient is that it only compares pairs of variables. There may be a very strong association between one variable and a *group* of others. This may not be reflected in any single correlation coefficient. (There are more sophisticated statistics which are used to investigate such associations.)

The correlation coefficient, sometimes called Pearson's correlation coefficient, is used to explore associations between two continuous variables. You may wish to explore associations between other pairs of variables (e.g. two ordinal variables, or an ordinal and a continuous variable). Different types of association require different methods. Again, it is important to understand the nature of the data.

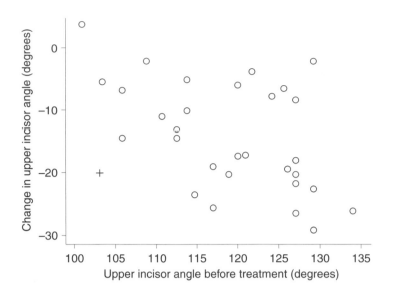

Figure 7.6 Scatter plot of the data shown in Figure 7.3, with one extra data point. The correlation coefficient is now –0.44, compared with –0.51.

Correlation does not imply causation

If there is a strong association between two variables, it may be that one is *influencing* the other. This would be evidence of causality. However, association does not imply causality. For example, there is a strong positive correlation between deaths by drowning and ice-cream sales. When many ice-creams are sold, more people die by drowning. You could not conclude that ice-cream causes drowning. What is the explanation? In fact, there is another variable which gives a better explanation – the temperature. When the temperature is high, more people buy ice-cream, but also when the temperature is high more people go to the beach and go swimming. The temperature is an example of what is sometimes called a *lurking variable*. There are many more apocryphal examples. For example:

- reading ability is associated with shoe size (lurking variable is age)
- general quality of health is associated with purchase of bottled water (lurking variable is socio-economic status).

For many years people used to try to argue that the association between smoking and cancer was non-causal; potential lurking variables were genetic make-up and socio-economic status.

Thus it is important to look out for lurking variables, and to remember that a causal relationship cannot be inferred from an observational study.

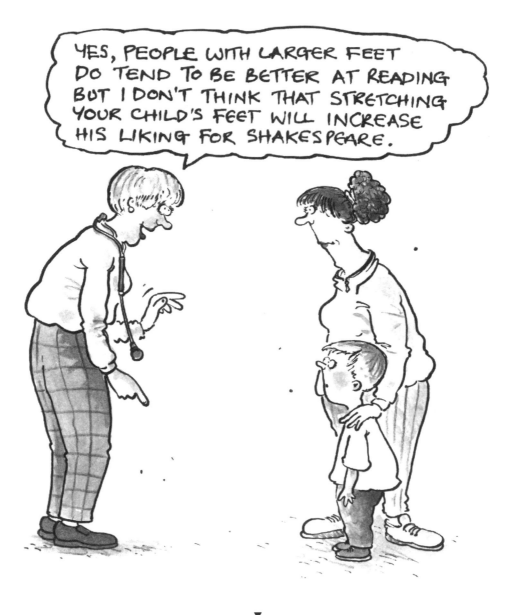

Correlation does not imply agreement

During the past few years there has been increasing interest in *reliability*. For example, you might be interested in comparing two instruments that are designed to measure the same quantity, or you might compare two people using the same instrument. In each case you would be interested in the degree to which the two sets of readings were in *agreement*. This idea can be extended to more than two sets of readings. A correlation coefficient is *not* a suitable statistic for this. Figure 7.7 illustrates the difference between correlation and agreement. The lines are artificial, but show plots of the readings of two observers observing exactly the same thing, and scoring the result on a scale of 1 to 7. The broken line shows perfect agreement – the value for observer 1 is always exactly the same as that for observer 2. There is clearly perfect correlation here, too. There is also perfect correlation for the solid line, but very little agreement. For the solid line, observer 2 almost always scores higher than observer 1, and the spread of scores is much lower. If there is high correlation but poor agreement between two measures or methods of measurement, a correction or *calibration* might be a feasible way of obtaining high agreement. This involves modelling the relationship between the two sets of values.

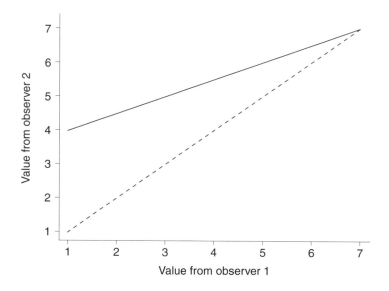

Figure 7.7 Correlation does not imply agreement. The solid line shows perfect correlation, but poor agreement, between the values from two observers. The broken line shows perfect agreement (and perfect correlation).

Agreement necessitates correlation, but correlation does not imply agreement. If you are comparing agreement between people who are using the same measure, correlation coefficients can be very misleading. Another statistic is needed, and intra-class correlations are used to measure agreement. When the responses are discrete or ordinal, the kappa statistic is suitable.[2,3]

Confounds

Relationships between variables can either be very useful or be a nuisance. It all depends on what you are trying to do. Consider the following example. Suppose you want to compare the efficacy of a treatment for which there is a suitable placebo. You recruit one set of subjects from one hospital and give them the treatment, and you recruit a second set of subjects from a second hospital and give them the placebo. You try to ensure that the age and gender profiles of the two groups are similar. At the end of the study there is a highly significant and important beneficial difference in the treatment group. However, you cannot validly attribute this difference to the treatment. Why not?

The difference in response or outcome could be attributable to any one or a set of the conditions which differ between the two groups. The treatment is only one of these. In addition:

- there are different doctors at the different hospitals
- there may be different levels of care at the two hospitals
- demographic characteristics might vary between the two groups
- the groups might have different socio-economic profiles
- the groups might have different severity of disease at the start of the study
- and so on ...

Any treatment effect is *confounded* with these other effects. It is impossible to tease out any specific treatment effect.

Published papers should report any possible confounds. An example is given in a study by Nyguyen and colleagues.[4] They conducted an RCT of spa therapy in comparison with the usual treatment for osteoarthritis. Spa therapy consisted of a 21-day period that included the journey, rest, balneotherapy, spring water and medical attention at the resort. The control group had a 21-day period during which the subjects maintained their routine care. The aim was to assess the carry-over symptomatic effect of 'spa therapy'. The authors state that:

> the inevitable more frequent contact of the spa patients with spa staff could also introduce a bias, since such contact could well result in additional explanation and education. Therefore such attention by spa medical staff could be considered as an individual component of the spa therapy which could contribute to improvement.

There are very many factors that differ between the two groups. These include the excitement of a trip, increased social contact, a change of geographical location and so on. These are all *confounds* for the effect of the spa waters.

Authors should, as in this example, identify possible confounds in the discussion of their results, but some are less self-critical than others. If you can think of possible confounds that have not been accounted for, you should treat the results with caution.

Interactions

Another way in which variables are associated is via *interactions*. Suppose you are studying the effect of a drug vs. placebo on the anxiety/depression score of individuals with depression. You have a suitably validated score, where a high value denotes high levels of anxiety/depression. It is possible that males and females might react differently to the drug. You set up a suitably designed study and measure the *percentage change* in score over the period of the study. Figures 7.8 to 7.10 show different types of results from such a study. Each plot shows the average percentage change for treatment and placebo groups, by gender. The values for the treatment groups are denoted by a plus sign. In Figure 7.8 both groups show an average percentage reduction in the score of about 50%. The difference between treatment and placebo is unlikely to be clinically significant, even if it is statistically significant. Similarly, there is little evidence of clinically significant differences between the sexes.

In Figure 7.9 the situation looks different. The plots show only the means, and give no idea of the *variability* of the results, so it is impossible to estimate the statistical significance from the figure. However, there is the suggestion

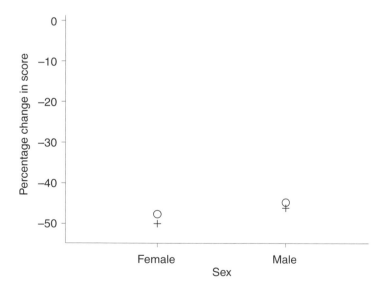

Figure 7.8   A plot of mean effects for treatment and placebo (+ represents treatment). There is no evidence of a difference between treatment and placebo, and little evidence of sex differences.

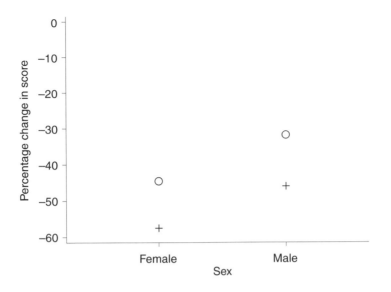

Figure 7.9 A plot of mean effects for treatment and placebo (+ represents treatment). There is evidence of a difference between treatment and placebo, and a sex difference. The differential effect of the treatment seems to be the same irrespective of sex.

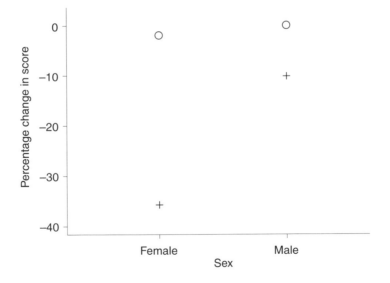

Figure 7.10 A plot of mean effects for treatment and placebo (+ represents treatment). The treatment effect seems to be more pronounced for females than for males.

of a difference between average treatment and placebo responses. For both groups there is an average improvement in scores (remember to look at the scale on the axes), but the treatment is associated with a greater average change. There is therefore evidence of a placebo effect, but also of a treatment effect. There is a suggestion that the percentage changes are greater in size for females than for males, but that the differential effect of the treatment is the same for each sex. There may be treatment and sex differences, but they are not related.

Figure 7.10 shows a case where there might be an *interaction*. This time the placebo has little overall effect on the scores (look at the scales). There is some evidence that the treatment reduces the average scores, and that this reduction is greater for females. Thus the average treatment effect for males is different from that for females – the effect is of the same type for each sex, but greater for females. This then is the interaction – the nature of the treatment effect depends on the sex. You cannot simply talk about a 'treatment effect' without reference to gender.

A different type of interaction is shown in Figure 7.11, which summarises the results obtained from a study comparing the effects of two different drugs. The mean effect of the new drug is denoted by a plus sign, and that for the standard drug is denoted by a circle. Here it is possible (if the results are statistically significant) that the new drug has opposite differential effects for the two sexes. For females the new drug has a much more pronounced

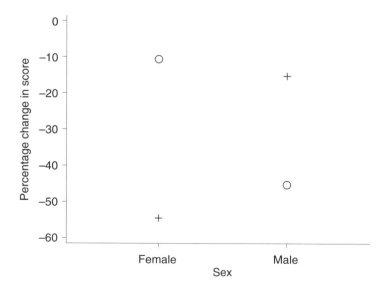

Figure 7.11   A plot of mean effects for a new drug (denoted by +) and a standard drug (denoted by O). The new drug appears to be more effective for females, but less effective for males.

average effect than does the standard drug (where the effect is relatively small). However, for males the greater average benefit is from the standard drug. Furthermore, note that for Figure 7.11, if you *ignore* gender there might appear to be little difference between the two treatments, and you could therefore fail to observe an interesting effect.

Interactions can therefore be extremely important. If there is good reason to suspect that there might be an important interactive effect, the study must be designed to be capable of detecting it. Note that where there is an interaction it can be difficult to describe any treatment effect without reference to the other factors with which it interacts. If an interaction has been found, the nature of that interaction should be described.

This section has not described all of the possible patterns of outcomes. What would the plots look like if there was a gender effect but no differential treatment effect? And what would they look like if there was a differential treatment effect but no gender effect?

Repeated measures

Another instance in which interactions are crucially important is where *repeated measures* are taken on the same individual. The simplest example of this is where a response is measured before treatment and after treatment – there are two measures per subject. One way to analyse such data is to compute the difference for each subject. However, it has already been noted that the change in response might be related – in fact *correlated* – with the initial baseline value. In repeated-measures studies, more than two measurements are taken on the same individual. Figures 7.12 to 7.15 show plots describing a study of two groups where measurements were taken on four occasions *at regular intervals*. The first was at baseline before any treatment, and there were three more measurement times during the study. The broken line shows the average responses for the treatment group, and the solid line shows those for the placebo group. Assume that a high score indicates something undesirable.

Since the measures on the same person are likely to be correlated (individuals with higher scores at the start are more likely to have higher scores at later times), the analysis must *model* the correlations. There are special methods for this. In Figure 7.12 the two plots look very similar. The average scores drop between assessments 1 and 2, but then seem to level off. If these effects were statistically significant, then this would be described as no group difference, but a time effect. How can this be explained? The effect is similar for both active treatment and placebo groups, so it could be a true placebo effect. On the other hand, it could be what is called an artefact – perhaps the subjects exaggerated their scores at the start of the study in order to ensure entry to a study which they thought might help them. Alternatively, the effect might be

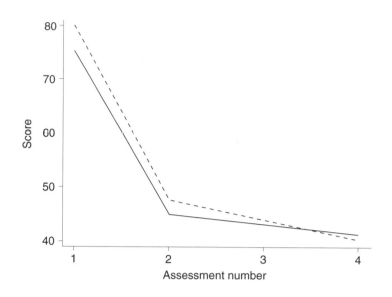

Figure 7.12   Results from a repeated-measures study. There seems to be a strong time effect, but no difference between the two groups.

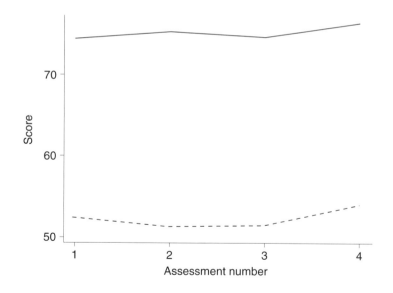

Figure 7.13   Results from a repeated-measures study. There is little evidence of a time effect, but there seems to be a group difference.

a consequence of the fact that patients with many conditions (especially related to bouts of depression) tend to improve over time – at least temporarily – without any treatment at all. Whatever the explanation, there is little

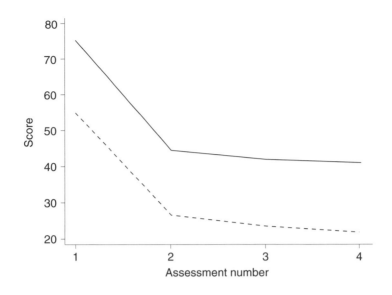

Figure 7.14 Results from a repeated-measures study. There is evidence of a time effect, and a group difference. The time effect looks the same for each group.

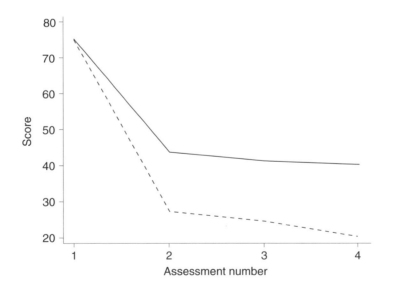

Figure 7.15 Results from a repeated-measures study. There is evidence of a time–group interaction. There is evidence of a time effect for each group, but the effect is different for each group.

evidence that the active treatment is better than placebo, although it may be that placebo has real benefits for the subjects.

Figure 7.13 shows two profiles where there is no evidence of a time effect. The profiles are almost flat. However, there seems to be a difference between the groups. Is this a differential treatment effect? The answer is that it cannot be. The first measurements are taken before any treatment commenced, and the average values do not appear to change. The differences are due to differences between the groups. Perhaps the randomisation process did not work very well, or perhaps you might expect such a degree of variability between two groups selected at random.

In Figure 7.14 there is the suggestion of both a group effect and a time effect. The time effect looks the same for each group. There is a drop in average scores from assessment 1 to assessment 2 and then a levelling off.

Figure 7.15 shows some evidence of a time–group interaction. Both groups start off with comparable average scores. The average scores drop between assessments 1 and 2 and then tend to level off, but the decrease for the treatment group looks larger. Even if there is a placebo effect, there seems to be a differential treatment effect which might be clinically significant.

Note that all of these descriptions make use of the fact that the assessments are made at *regular intervals*. Had the assessments been made at irregular intervals, the plots of mean score against assessment number could have been misleading. Plots against actual assessment times might have been better, and the patterns and resulting interpretations could have been different. Remember to look carefully at the scales on graphs.

These examples show how repeated measures can give a deeper insight into what has happened in a study. Think how the conclusions would be weaker if only the 'before' and 'after' responses had been measured in these cases. However, there is another reason for taking repeated measures. It is a way of increasing the *power* of a study. It can be costly and difficult to recruit large numbers of subjects. Obviously it costs more to take more measurements, but it may be more practical than requiring many more subjects. However, problems can occur if subjects fail to attend all of the assessments. Issues such as this need to be discussed during the design stage.

A very common mistake is to take repeated measures on the same subjects, but to treat the data as if they were *independent*. Two variables are independent if knowing about the value of one of them tells you nothing about the other one. Random samples generate independent values, because the values are chosen at random, and the choice of one item does not affect whether or not another one is chosen. However, if you take six people and measure their pain thresholds at ten different parts of their bodies, you do not have 60 independent values. Someone with a low threshold at one location is likely to have a low threshold at the other locations. This must be modelled in the analysis. You would have 60 independent values if you randomly selected 60 people and took one reading from each of them (ideally at the same location, if you wanted to combine the results). Similarly, if four therapists each rate five patients, the analysis must take into account the fact that the same therapists are making repeated diagnoses. Repeated measures are not independent.

In practice, care must be taken in analysing repeated measures. Specifically, it is important to treat any measures made before treatment correctly. It is a good idea to consult an expert.

Summary

Associations may exist between different variables. Associations need careful description and interpretation. Key points include the following.

- A straight line is an example of a simple model of an association between two variables.
- The correlation coefficient measures the degree of linear association between two continuous variables, but it can be very sensitive to a few atypical data points.
- Correlation does not imply causation or agreement.
- An interaction occurs when the effect of one variable is influenced by the value of another variable.
- Repeated measures produce data in which the values from the same subject are correlated.

CHAPTER EIGHT

Where is the evidence?

Any professional would want to give the most up-to-date and appropriate advice. Sadly, however, much medical practice is not supported by sound science. Part of the problem is the sheer volume of published material, much of which describes methodologically flawed studies.[1,2] The problem is therefore to access the relevant material without having to plough through the irrelevant.

This chapter will give advice on the following:

- the *hierarchy* of evidence – what are the best-quality studies?
- how to read a paper critically
- the outcome measures most commonly used in evidence-based medicine.

This chapter contains some formulae. These are included because they are so fundamental to evidence-based medicine.

The hierarchy of evidence

Chapter 1 discussed different types of study design. The randomised controlled trial (RCT) is regarded as the most rigorous and methodologically pure method for evaluation of therapies, especially if it is double-blind. As a general rule, therefore, the results of an RCT will be of more value than, for example, a cohort study. Unfortunately, there are both well-designed clinical trials and badly designed ones. The value of a study depends not only on the type of design, but also on its size and overall quality. A good cohort study could be of more value than a poor clinical trial. For the moment, assume that you are comparing high-quality studies. There is a commonly accepted hierarchy of evidence, which is shown in Figure 8.1.

Belief and anecdote cannot really qualify as 'evidence', although they might form the basis for a research question and so motivate one of the studies in the triangle. The types of study that are higher in the triangle are experimental as opposed to observational. In experiments, groups of subjects

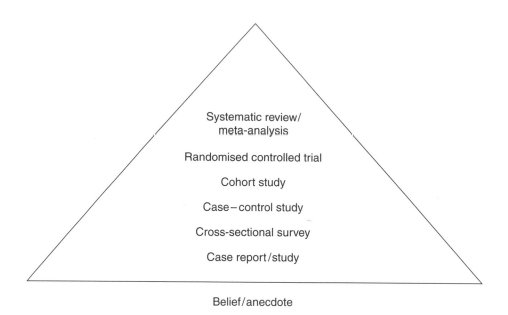

Figure 8.1   The hierarchy of evidence. The higher the study is in the triangle, the better the quality of evidence. Belief and anecdote do not qualify as evidence.

are more likely to be comparable prior to any intervention, data are collected prospectively and so are more reliable, and the allocation of 'treatment' is more under the experimenter's control. This reduces the effects of confounding, and makes it much easier to demonstrate causal links.

The high-quality systematic review and meta-analysis lie right at the top of the triangle, and provide the strongest evidence. Each of these studies involves combining the results from other published (or even unpublished) studies. A review is a survey of studies. The problem with this is that you can select papers that agree with your own personal view and ignore those with which you disagree. In this way you might be able to put together a beguiling argument for your case. However, it would be both biased and unscientific. In a *systematic review* a specific research question is posed, and the reviewer searches systematically for *all* studies which have addressed this question. This search has to be as comprehensive as possible, and the search methods should be stated. The studies are then rated according to explicitly stated quality criteria. Sets of criteria are generally more useful than scoring systems, most of which are not adequately validated. Some studies may be excluded from the subsequent analysis if they do not meet the quality criteria. The paper then summarises the totality of evidence provided by the studies. A good systematic review will give you a wealth of information about a particular research question. Remember to look at the date of the paper.

A *meta-analysis* combines the results of several studies to give, for example, a single confidence interval for a therapeutic effect. Such papers usually report the confidence intervals of each of the contributing studies, and state how the combined result has been obtained. As you might expect, the resulting confidence interval tends to be narrower than the individual ones. The method can also be useful for combining the results of studies whose results have been 'marginal' with those which appeared to give a more definite result.

A systematic review can contain a meta-analysis, but need not do so. Similarly, a meta-analysis may or may not be based on a systematic review. You need to read papers carefully in order to determine exactly which type you have found.

Typical questions addressed by these studies include the following.

- What is the evidence from RCTs for the efficacy of acupuncture in the treatment of neck pain?[3]
- What is the evidence for the efficacy of treatments for the painful heel?[4]
- What is the effectiveness of routine ultrasound scanning in pregnancy?[5]

Systematic reviews and meta-analyses can be extremely useful, if sometimes difficult to read. None the less, a good large RCT can be of greater value than either a mediocre systematic review, or a good systematic review of poor-quality studies. Similarly, a large-scale, multicentre, well-designed RCT can be of much more value than a meta-analysis of many observational studies.

Causality

The RCT is methodologically 'pure' because, as discussed in Chapter 1, a well-designed RCT can establish *causal* links as opposed to mere association. However, RCTs are not always possible, and good observational studies are then the best approach. An important question arises. When is the information from a study of high enough quality for you to be able to infer a causal relationship between, say, a risk factor and a disease? Sir Austin Bradford Hill addressed this question many years ago. The presence of the following conditions strengthens the case for causality.[6]

- There is strong evidence of a *strong* association between the risk factor and the disease.
- Exposure to the risk factor occurred *before* the disease onset.
- There is a biological *explanation* for the causal relationship.
- The evidence for the association should come from *several studies* in a variety of settings.
- There should be evidence of a *dose–response* effect – if the risk factor is eliminated, the likelihood of the disease should be eliminated or reduced.

Similarly, if the amount of exposure to the risk factor is increased, the likelihood of the disease should also be increased.

- There is *no* other credible explanation (e.g. confounding).

These principles can be generalised to other observational studies. You should bear them in mind when evaluating the quality of an observational study.

Evaluating the literature

It is essential to search wisely for material and to read critically. A first indication of the quality of material is its source. Although there is a wealth of useful information on the Internet, there is no peer review process, and consequently there is no validity check of material. Books are generally of better quality because they are subjected to an editorial process, but this may not involve peer review. Moreover, they rapidly become dated. Journals have peer review, but the strictness of the process varies tremendously from one journal to another. There is intense pressure to publish, and editors of some of the less prestigious journals do not apply rigid standards. Of course, this does not mean that there is nothing of value on the Internet or in the less prestigious journals. For example, the *British Medical Journal* web-page (www.bmj.com) is an excellent source of material, including the *BMJ* online.

While you may have your 'favourite' journal, it is likely that material relevant to you is published in many places. You will not have the time to search them all. However, all is not lost. While the advent of computers has caused an explosion in the volume of material, it has also facilitated mechanisms to allow you to access that material in an efficient manner. The obvious mechanism is by online searches using a database such as Medline,[7] and there is an increasing number of online journals. The number of database facilities is also increasing. The Cochrane Library (update.cochrane.co.uk) provides high-quality systematic reviews of trials, and is a very valuable source of information. There is also a wealth of 'evidence-based' material in journals and online. Journals such as *Evidence-Based Medicine* summarise the published material. Experts search the general literature and select quality studies for the journal. The selected papers are summarised and commented on. In other words, someone else does the searching for you. Facilities like this are also appearing online, for example *Best Evidence*. Full details cannot be given here (as the information would become out of date immediately), but there are excellent sources of information.[8]

Notwithstanding all of these facilities, you are still likely to end up reading a paper for yourself and critically evaluating it. You should *always* read critically. Reviewers are human, and even the best journals publish papers containing flaws or mistakes. It is not sufficient merely to read the introduction and conclusions and then to use them to inform clinical practice. Nor should you simply count the number of papers that endorse a particular view. It is quality, not just quantity, that counts.

There are specific criteria for evaluating different types of studies. For example, the CONSORT statement is increasingly being adopted to ensure the quality of papers that report RCTs.[9]

The following advice is fairly generic, and is a starting point for *any* paper, including review articles.

Most papers follow the IMRAD format – Introduction, Methods, Results And Discussion. To avoid wasting time, the first section to concentrate on is the Methods section. The principle of Garbage In, Garbage Out applies here. If a study is badly designed it cannot address the research question, and the results – however impressive the confidence intervals, sophisticated modelling or *P*-values – are not worth reading. The following questions then form a starting point for evaluation.

- What was the research question?
- Is the study described fully? Is enough information provided for you to be able to repeat it?
- How did the researchers take into account what was already known about the subject?
- What does this study add to what is already known about the subject?
- Does the study design match the question?
- What is the study population?
- Was a sample-size calculation made to try to ensure that any relevant effect had a good chance of being detected?
- Who were the subjects?
    Are they typical of the study population?
    How were they recruited?
    Who was excluded/included?
    Is there any bias?
- Was randomisation adequate?
- Was concealment adequate?
- What was the outcome measure?
    Why was it chosen?
    Was it suitable?
    Was it validated?
- Were the subjects/assessors blinded where possible?
- Are the data described fully?
- Are odd/interesting cases or outliers described?
    Are they dealt with in a suitable manner?
- How are dropouts dealt with?

- Is the statistical analysis appropriate?
- Are confidence intervals given for main effects?
- Are exact *P*-values given?
- Does the paper discuss the *clinical* relevance of the results?
- Does the paper discuss the limitations of the study?
- Are possible confounds discussed satisfactorily?
- Can the results be generalised to your situation?

Similar lists and advice are given in other sources.[10–13]

If you are not satisfied with the answer to any such question that you believe to be important, then the lesson is clear – treat the conclusions of the paper with caution. Remember, however, that the absence of evidence is not evidence of absence. Journals often impose word limits on papers, and authors therefore have to be selective in what they report. Thus you cannot be sure that a feature was absent from a study just because the authors have not reported it. (This is a problem that has to be faced by researchers carrying out systematic reviews.) None the less, the authors will have described what they consider to be the most important features of their study. Moreover, no study is perfect, and it is easy to be wise 'after the event'. Authors should therefore be self-critical of their results.

Examples

Throughout this book reference has been made to a number of published studies. Other texts give examples of how to carry out detailed evaluations of papers,[14] and it is not my aim to do so here. However, for each of the research papers used in this book, here are some specific questions that you might well ask. Of course, you should always ask the questions in the list above. You should also think of questions that *you* personally would ask of these studies. If you can get hold of the papers you should be able to answer them.

Case Study A – nurse consultation system[15]

- Are the outcome measures appropriate and sufficient?
- Which time periods does the study cover?
- Was the blinding adequate?
- How typical is the general practice co-operative?
- How typical are the patients in this area?

- What were the specific conditions?
    - Training of nurses?
    - Technology used?
- How general are the findings?

Case Study B – postnatal catch-up[16]

- Where was the study carried out?
- Which infants were included/excluded?
- How general are the findings?

Case Study C – survey of doctors in Norway[17]

- Was the study supposed to be a census or a survey?
- Can the results be generalised to other countries/years?
- Was the response rate high enough to minimise bias?
- Was the questionnaire valid?
- Could the questionnaire be used elsewhere?

Case Study D – effect of TV programme on overdose attempts[18]

- Is the design appropriate (the answer is probably 'yes')?
- Did they ask the most relevant questions?
- Were the periods studied long enough?
- Were the hospitals included 'representative'?
- What are the general conclusions?

Terms used in evidence-based medicine

This is the section that contains some equations. So far relatively simple summary statistics have been described. Evidence-based medicine has its own terminology, and it is important that you understand it. (More details and examples are given elsewhere.[8,10])

First of all, consider the situation where there are two groups – an experimental (treatment) group and a control group. Suppose that the treatment is designed to *reduce the risk of an adverse event*. For example, the treatment could be aspirin and the adverse event could be myocardial infarct.

The following definitions are used.

CER is the *control event rate* (the rate at which the event occurs in the control group).

EER is the *experimental event rate* (the rate at which the event occurs in the treatment group).

These rates are often expressed as percentages. So if the CER is 12% and the EER is 2%, we can say that:

- 12% of subjects in the control group experience the adverse event
- 2% of subjects in the treatment group experience the adverse event.

The following definitions are also used.

ARR is the *absolute risk reduction*. ARR = CER − EER. This is also a percentage. It is the simple difference in percentages between the two groups. In this example, ARR = 10%. The treatment reduces the rate of adverse events by 10 percentage points.

However, the ARR takes no account of the rate in the control group – it is simply the difference. The relative risk reduction (RRR) gives this difference as a percentage of the rate that you expect in the control group.

RRR is the *relative risk reduction*. RRR = (CER − EER)/CER, or equivalently RRR = ARR/CER. It is expressed as a percentage. In this example RRR = 10/12 = 83%. A large proportion of the risk appears to be removed by the treatment.

NNT is the *number needed to treat*. This is the number of patients you would expect to need to treat in order to avoid *one* adverse event.

Here:

- for 100 patients in the control group you expect 12 adverse events
- for 100 patients treated you expect two adverse events
- if you treat 100 patients you avoid 12−2 = 10 adverse events
- if you treat 10 patients you avoid one adverse event.

So here the NNT is 10. This means that for every 10 patients you treat, you expect to avoid one adverse event.

There is a formula that gives you the NNT directly. There are two steps:

1 Calculate 1/ARR.
2 If the answer is not a whole number, round it *up*. The answer is the NNT.

Here is another example:

CER = 27%
EER = 13%.
Then ARR = 27% – 13% = 14%.
RRR = 14/27 = 52%
and 1/ARR = 1/(14%) = 7.14.
So NNT = 8.

Note here that the absolute risk reduction is higher than that in the previous example, so the number needed to treat is lower. However, the relative risk reduction is much lower, because the rate of events in the control group is higher initially. The various statistics tell you different things, which is why it is important to understand them. Measures such as this do not take into account the costs of treatment, but they are used in economic analyses.

(At this point you may well ask, 'What about confidence intervals?'. You would be right – these statistics should be accompanied by confidence intervals. However, for simplicity they are omitted here.)

The treatment might not be intended to decrease the risk of an adverse event. It could be designed to increase the likelihood of a beneficial event, or the treatment could actually increase the likelihood of an adverse event. It would not be intended to achieve the latter, of course. Similar statistics exist for these other two cases. They are summarised in Table 8.1.

Table 8.1   Summary of terms used in evidence-based medicine

Treatment reduces likelihood of an adverse event			
ARR	Absolute risk reduction	CER – EER	(percentage)
RRR	Relative risk reduction	(CER – EER)/CER	(percentage)
NNT	Number needed to treat	1/ARR (rounded up)	(number)
Treatment increases likelihood of a desirable event			
ABI	Absolute benefit increase	EER – CER	(percentage)
RBI	Relative benefit increase	(EER – CER)/CER	(percentage)
NNT	Number needed to treat	1/ABI (rounded up)	(number)
Treatment increases likelihood of an adverse event			
ARI	Absolute risk increase	EER – CER	(percentage)
RRI	Relative risk increase	(EER – CER)/CER	(percentage)
NNH	Number needed to harm	1/ARI (rounded up)	(number)

Another term you are likely to encounter, especially in systematic reviews, is the *odds ratio*. This is best introduced via the *relative risk*.

Consider the artificial data shown in Table 8.2, obtained from a prospective study. There are two groups – a control group and a treatment group.

Table 8.2   Example of data used to calculate an odds ratio

	Event occurs	*Event does not occur*	*Total*
Treatment	7	93	100
No treatment (control)	3	147	150

Seven of the 100 subjects in the treatment group experience an event, compared to three of the 150 subjects in the control group.

- The risk of the event for the treatment group is $7/100 = 7\%$.
- The risk of the event for the control group is $3/150 = 2\%$.

The relative risk of the event is a ratio of the two risks. Here it is $7/2 = 3.5$. Note that this is a number, not a percentage. In other words, the event is 3.5 times more likely to occur in the treatment group than in the control group.

For the more general case illustrated in Table 8.3:

$$\text{Relative risk RR} = (a/(a + b))/(c/(c + d)).$$

This can be written as:

$$\text{RR} = \frac{a(c + d)}{c(a + b)}.$$

Table 8.3   General format for calculating an odds ratio

	Event occurs	*Event does not occur*	*Total*
Treatment	a	b	$a + b$
No treatment (control)	c	d	$c + d$

The value for 'no effect' is 1. So:

- $\text{RR} = 1$ means risk factor *not associated* with the event
- $\text{RR} > 1$ means risk factor associated with *increased* likelihood of the event
- $\text{RR} < 1$ means risk factor associated with *decreased* likelihood of the event.

Now the *odds* (used mostly by gamblers) are as follows.

- The odds of the event in the treatment group are $7/93$ or a/b.
- The odds of the event in the control group are $3/147$ or c/d.

The *odds ratio* is the ratio of the two sets of odds – that is, 3.7 or $(ad)/(bc)$.

In this example, the odds ratio is of similar size to the relative risk. It defines the odds of a patient in the treatment group experiencing the event, relative to a patient in the control group. The odds ratio will be similar to the relative risk *when the event rates are low*. In such cases the odds ratio is often used as an approximation for the relative risk.

Here is an example.

Table 8.4   Example of data used to calculate an odds ratio. Here the event rates are high, so the odds ratio cannot be used to approximate the relative risk

	Event occurs	*Event does not occur*	*Total*
Treatment	60	40	100
No treatment (control)	70	80	150

The relative risk is 1.29.

The odds ratio is 1.71.

Here the event rates arc high (the risks are 60% and 47%), so the odds ratio *cannot* be used to approximate the relative risk.

You will also see the odds ratio in reports of case–control studies. It is often estimated in a modelling process known as *logistic regression*. This is a special type of regression that models the *probabilities* that events of interest will occur. However, the interpretation of the odds ratios is just the same. A case–control study is a retrospective study in which individuals are selected because of the *event*, not because of the treatment (or exposure). The number of events is therefore not representative of the proportion in the population. This means that it is impossible to estimate risks, but the odds ratio is still valid.

For example, a group of researchers investigated the link between exposure to sunlight and deaths from multiple sclerosis.[19] The data were drawn from death certificates.

Exposure to sunlight was determined by the place of residence of the person, using only individuals who had lived in a particular region all of their life. The researchers found 4282 cases of death from multiple sclerosis and 115 195 controls. The data are shown in Table 8.5.

Table 8.5   Data from a case–control study of deaths from multiple sclerosis and exposure to sunlight

	Multiple sclerosis	*Controls*
High exposure to sunlight	919	31 247
Moderate exposure to sunlight	1552	50 252
Low exposure to sunlight	1811	33 696
Total	4282	115 195

In the paper, the odds ratio (95% confidence interval) for high exposure to sunlight relative to low exposure is 0.55 (0.51 to 0.59), and that for moderate exposure compared to low exposure is 0.58 (0.54 to 0.62). The authors conclude that 'residential ... solar radiation [is] inversely associated with mortality from multiple sclerosis'.

The odds ratio *is less than one*, so exposure to sunlight is associated with a *lower likelihood* of death from multiple sclerosis. This is what is meant by 'inversely' related. Note that the confidence intervals do not contain the 'no effect' value of one. So there is evidence of an association between exposure to sunlight and death from multiple sclerosis. We need to be assured that there are no confounding or lurking variables before we can define this as a causal relationship.

Another situation in which you might be presented with a table of counts is in a study about a diagnostic test. Suppose there is a test that is intended to identify patients with a particular disease. The result of a test can be either positive or negative – the person either has the disease or does not have it. It is assumed that there is some gold-standard method that establishes the 'truth'.

Table 8.6 shows a format for analysing the quality of the test. Ideally you want the numbers b and c to be zero. This is because the box containing b describes cases where the test is positive, but the patient does not have the disease. These are *false-positive* cases. The box containing d describes *false-negative* cases, where the person does have the disease, but the test is negative. This is very similar to the various outcomes in hypothesis testing.

Table 8.6   Example of data describing the quality of a diagnostic test

	Disease present	*Disease not present*
Positive test result	a	b
Negative test result	c	d

The following definitions are often used.

- The *prevalence* of the disease for this sample is $(a + c)/(a + b + c + d)$.
- The *positive prediction* (or *predictive*) *rate* is $a/(a + b)$. It is the likelihood that a person who tests positive actually has the disease.
- The *negative prediction rate* is $d/(c + d)$. It is the likelihood that a person who tests negative does not have the disease.
- The *sensitivity* of the test is $a/(a + c)$. It is the likelihood that a person who has the disease tests positive.

- The *specificity* of the test is $d/(b + d)$. It is the likelihood that a person who does not have the disease tests negative.
- The overall *accuracy* of the test is $(a + d)/(a + b + c + d)$.

Sensitivity and *specificity* are the most commonly used terms. Ideally you want high values (close to one) for both. However, as with hypothesis tests, in general this is difficult to achieve. Tests often have a threshold for making a decision – 'decide yes if the score exceeds the threshold value'. You can set the threshold to obtain high specificity, but this might be at the risk of lower sensitivity, and vice versa. The 'best' threshold depends on the clinical setting, especially on the risks associated with the wrong decisions.

General rules of thumb are as follows.

- If a test has *high specificity*, then a *positive* test result means that you probably *do* have the disease.
- If a test has *high sensitivity*, then a *negative* test result means that you probably do *not* have the disease.
- If a test has both *high sensitivity and high specificity*, then a *positive* test result means that you probably *do* have the disease and a *negative* result means that you probably *do not* have the disease.

For practical purposes it is the positive and negative prediction rates that are of most clinical relevance. However, these values depend on the *prevalence* of the disease, and are therefore very dependent on the composition of the sample. Typically, if there is a disproportionate number of diseased cases in the sample, this will affect the prediction rates, whereas it will not affect the sensitivity and specificity. Therefore you should never regard predictive rates obtained from a sample as generally applicable.

Sometimes people use the sensitivity and specificity to produce a *receiver operating characteristic (ROC)* curve. This is a plot of sensitivity against (1 – specificity). For an ideal test you want both values to be close to 1, which means (1 – specificity) close to zero. Figure 8.2 shows two ROC curves. The broken line describes a good test – it has high specificity and high sensitivity. On the other hand, the solid line describes a test that is not good. It lies close to the diagonal line from the bottom left-hand corner to the top right-hand corner, which is the line corresponding to guesswork. A test with an ROC curve like the solid one is not much better than tossing a coin.

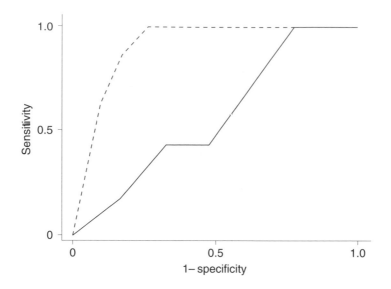

Figure 8.2   Two ROC curves. The broken line denotes a good test, and the solid line denotes a poor one.

Summary

- There is a hierarchy of evidence, but you should take into account the quality of a study as well as its type.
- Evidence databases are a good source of information.
- Always read papers critically.
- Make sure that you are familiar with the terms used in evidence-based medicine.

CHAPTER NINE

Liaising with a statistician

If your only encounter with statistics is when you read published papers, this chapter may be of limited interest to you. It is intended for researchers who need to liaise with a statistician. After reading the chapter you should have a better idea about:

- what statisticians do
- how to liaise with them.

General advice

Statisticians are like apples, bananas and healthcare studies – some are better than others. However, involving a good statistician in all aspects of your statistical work can only improve its quality. First of all, find out who is your local statistician and their relationship with you. You may have an in-house statistician or an arrangement with a local university. They may have advertised surgery times or be available all day by telephone. Who pays them? What sort of help are you entitled to? Will they be an adviser or a collaborator?

Try to appreciate what they do. If you do not want to annoy a statistician, avoid making one of the following comments.

- 'It's a very simple question – it won't take you long to work it out.'
- 'We've done the study and submitted an abstract for a meeting. We just need someone to do the analysis.'
- 'I don't really want to discuss that. Can't you just tell me the sample size I need?'
- 'You're just the person I need. I've done a study on pain after operation. I've collected data from patients about how bad they feel the pain is after the operation. I didn't ask them about the pain beforehand. What values should I put in?'
- 'I've got some output here, but I don't really understand the method. Can you tell me what it means if I read it out over the phone?'

- 'You will input all the data, won't you?'
- 'I didn't expect to discuss ethical issues with you. I'm happy with the design.'
- 'I don't know which keys to press, but I know that's what you're good at.'

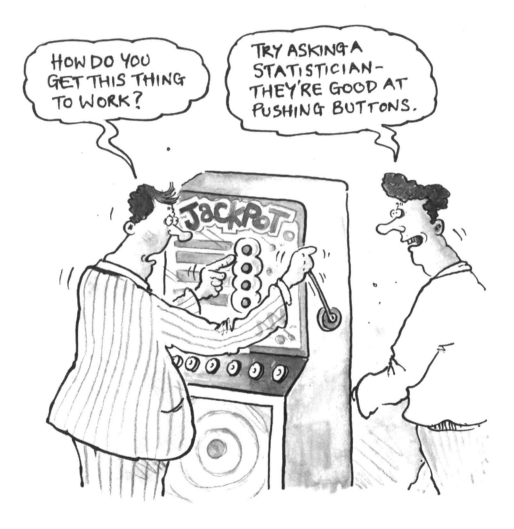

Things that statisticians do

What do *you* think statisticians do? Most people seem to think that they 'analyse data'. Worse still, some imagine this to be a simple matter of just hitting the right keys on a computer.

Statisticians are scientists who deal with all aspects of experiments and studies designed to collect numerical data. This book has emphasised the importance of study *design*. It should come as little surprise, therefore, to learn that statisticians play a major role in design. More than that, they strongly prefer to be involved in a study from the very early stages. A poor design cannot be redeemed by a clever analysis – prevention is much better than cure. In fact, it is fairly common for a statistician to spend more time discussing and refining the design than working on the analysis. This can be a creative process that is not highly structured, but it is worth all the effort. It involves discussion about the research question, outcome measures, predictor variables, confounds and lurking variables, samples and sample sizes. The design might change several times during this process, until you end up with a design which both matches a useful question and is feasible. You may wish to talk to other people, and so may your statistician. You should not expect a 'quick solution' at this stage.

Statisticians therefore help in the critical stage of designing a study. They are also helpful in a number of other ways.

- They often serve on ethics committees, or are accustomed to evaluating study protocols. They can help you to put together a protocol.
- They give advice on running a project. This involves preventing bad practice such as looking at data prematurely. They can predict some of the things that are likely to go wrong, and they can advise on how to collect and record data. This includes advice on how to design a database or spreadsheet, how to name variables and how to code missing values.
- They can give advice and training on the use of software packages for data entry and analysis. They can also advise on methods of analysis.
- They model data. By now you know that this means much more than just carrying out a test in order to obtain a *P*-value. Different types of data require different models. It is unethical to collect a large amount of data and to use only a small amount of it in the analysis. A statistician should be able to choose a suitable model for obtaining the maximum amount of information from the data without cheating or data dredging. As was discussed in Chapter 7, this is a complex process which involves a lot of model checking.
- They are good at qualitative reasoning. This means discussing the results and their implications. It is not a simple matter of judging whether something is significant or not significant.
- They help to present results and to write papers, and they can interpret the findings of other publications.

Do's and Don'ts

Below are some general tips.

Do:

- choose a statistician with a good reputation
- agree on the ground rules early on (e.g. who owns the data, and who will do what)
- think about where you are going to meet
- give your statistician time to think about the study
- be prepared to explain/describe/elucidate/go over matters in more detail
- be prepared to answer questions even if you cannot see their immediate relevance
- ask for clarification of terms that you do not understand
- be prepared to consider other designs
- ask about anything you are not sure about
- be prepared to let them see papers of previous studies
- be prepared to show them any apparatus or equipment to be used
- be prepared to justify your use of a tool or an outcome measure
- be prepared to check data values that look odd
- discuss alternative interpretations of the data
- discuss odd observations
- record all information, including dropouts and missing values
- treat the statistician as a fellow scientist.

Do not:

- expect to do everything by telephone
- expect an immediate reply
- assume that the statistician will understand everything you are talking about
- take criticism of your design personally.

Size of study

Your study needs to be large enough to have a reasonable chance of detecting the effect or difference of interest if it is really there. At the same time, it should not be too large, as this might involve a waste of resources or putting patients at unnecessary risk.

'Power calculation' is the name given to the process of deciding on the size of a study.

Before this you are likely to be asked the following questions.

- What is the specific research question and why is it important?
- What is already known?
- What is the precise effect that you are trying to find or estimate?
- What is your primary outcome measure, and what type of data will it generate?
- What variables are likely to influence this outcome measure?
- What instrument will you use to measure it? Is it valid?
- How easy is it to recruit subjects?
- What could go wrong?

Then, specifically for the power calculation, you are likely to be asked about the following:

- the expected response in the control group
- the size of a clinically relevant effect
- the variability of the outcome measure
- the relative sizes of different groups (do you want equal-sized groups?).

If you have secondary outcome measures, you may need to answer the second set of questions for each of these, too.

You may then need to estimate non-completion rates, because the power calculation relates to completers.

Finally ...

It is disappointing to read comments like the following:

> One of the drawbacks of this approach is that it involves statistical modelling. Expert statistical help is therefore required .... However, the economic and ethical advantages make it well worth facing the problem of statistical advice.

If research is worth doing, it is worth doing well. Where it involves human subjects it is unethical not to use the most appropriate methods. If you do have access to a statistician, *please* ask for their involvement as soon as possible, and work together as a team. If the statistician has the time, the ideal situation is for them to be a true collaborator – a co-owner of all aspects of the study. Research is 90% drudgery and 10% excitement, but the 10% is truly worth all of the effort.

Summary

- Statisticians can advise on all stages of quantitative research.
- They prefer to be involved from the start, especially in the design.
- They should be treated as collaborators.

APPENDIX A

Simple randomisation

Suppose that you want to recruit 50 subjects and to allocate them randomly to one of two groups. Normally the subjects do not all present themselves at the same time, so the allocation has to be done as and when a subject enters the study, *after* they have been recruited, been checked for eligibility and given their consent.

A series of random numbers is given below. They have been generated by a computer, and at any stage any of the numbers 0 to 9 is equally likely to occur.

7498**23053424**4569**3941**6298**205**46**0448**307
98853**7400**5770**8**26367101679831614002438**7**

Here is a suitable rule:

If the next random number is 0, 1, 2, 3 or 4, allocate the next subject to group A. Otherwise allocate the subject to group B.

The numbers relating to group A have been highlighted above. In practice this list is not available for inspection. Typically, a set of numbered, sealed, opaque envelopes is produced, each containing the group allocation for that subject.

Below are the first 12 envelopes. Remember that in practice you would not be able to see inside them.

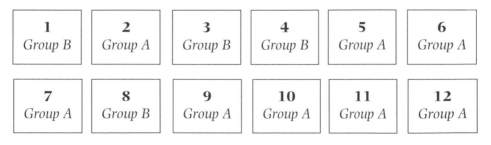

| 1 | 2 | 3 | 4 | 5 | 6 |
| Group B | Group A | Group B | Group B | Group A | Group A |

| 7 | 8 | 9 | 10 | 11 | 12 |
| Group A | Group B | Group A | Group A | Group A | Group A |

The subjects now start to arrive ...

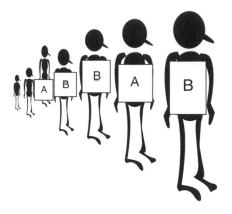

The first subject arrives. The envelope is opened and the person is allocated to group B. The second person is allocated to group A, the third is allocated to group B, and so on.

Notice that after 12 subjects have entered the study, there are only 4 subjects in group B and 8 subjects in group A. This has happened by chance. After 50 subjects have been recruited, 26 individuals will have been allocated to group A and 24 individuals to group B – the numbers are more equal. For small studies the process might be modified to ensure more equal numbers in groups. It can also be modified to try to obtain groups that are balanced with regard to other important characteristics.

APPENDIX B

Selecting a random sample from a sampling frame

Suppose that we have a list of 40 people and we want to select a simple random sample of 5 subjects. First of all we list the 40 subjects and give them unique labels 01–40 as follows.

01	Rebekah	11	Chris	21	**Mandy**	31	Barbara
02	James	12	Eddie	22	Debbie	32	Gordon
03	Anna	13	Paul	23	Karen	33	Victor
04	Phil	14	Judith	24	Bill	34	Susie
05	**Heather**	15	Mary	25	Khaleel	35	Zachary
06	**Luke**	16	Kathryn	26	**Valerie**	36	Edna
07	John	17	Simon	27	Shabnam	37	Joan
08	Margaret	18	Maria	28	Ryan	38	Stan
09	Joseph	19	Lesley	29	Rachel	39	Adrian
10	David	20	**Azim**	30	Ronald	40	Edzard

Then we generate a series of random numbers from a computer. They are digits 0–9, and at any stage each of them is equally likely to appear. We divide them into successive pairs as follows:

52,49,55,86,59,<u>06</u>,99,43,<u>26</u>,72,<u>20</u>,<u>05</u>,65,80,75
71,<u>21</u>,14,39,21,72,56,14,33,75,30,80,91,85

Now we go along the list selecting codes that are in the range 01 to 40. The first is 06, so Luke is selected. The next is 26, so Valerie is selected, and so on.

At the end of this process, our random selection of five people consists of Luke, Valerie, Azim, Heather and Mandy.

We have two males and three females. If we wanted two samples of equal size – one of males and the other of females – we would have to modify this basic process.

Glossary of terms

This is a glossary of the terms you are most likely to encounter. Some of the definitions are rather 'informal'. More precise, detailed or advanced information is given elsewhere.[1–3]

allocation concealment the process whereby the people recruiting subjects to a trial are blinded to the treatment group to which those subjects will be assigned. This is important in order to eliminate selection bias.

alternative hypothesis in hypothesis testing, this hypothesis will be 'accepted' when the null hypothesis is rejected. Often the alternative hypothesis is the one in which you are really interested.

ARR absolute risk reduction – the difference in rates of an undesirable event between the control and experimental groups. It is a percentage value.

assumptions the conditions required by a parametric test in order for its results to be valid.

balanced a study of two groups is said to be balanced with respect to a particular variable if the distribution of that variable is similar in the two groups.

bar chart a chart showing the frequencies of the values of a nominal variable. The bars are generally separated, and their lengths are proportional to the frequencies.

baseline measure a measure of some characteristic that is recorded for subjects at the start of a study, before any treatment commences.

bias a systematic error that leads to results which are consistently either too large or too small.

binary a binary variable can take one of two values (e.g. true/false).

boxplot a chart that is often used to compare two or more samples of ordinal or continuous variables. A boxplot shows the median, lower and upper quartiles, the maximum and minimum values, and possible outliers.

calibration the process of finding the relationship between two scales or instruments that measure the same thing.

case–control study an observational study designed to find relationships between, for example, a risk factor and a disease. A group of cases (with the disease) are compared with a group of controls (without the disease) with regard to their exposure to the risk factor. The data are summarised by an odds ratio.

case report published details of a clinical case history.

case series the results of a series of cases.

censored censored data often occur in studies of survival data. The data are censored if the event has not been observed during the duration of the study.

census a survey of an entire population.

central limit theorem a theorem which tells you about the distribution of the sample mean of large samples. For large samples, the sample mean is normally distributed.

CER control event rate – the rate at which a particular event occurs in the control group. It is a percentage.

cohort a group of subjects who share some characteristic in common, which is studied over time.

confidence interval a range of values, based on data from a sample, when you are attempting to estimate the parameter of a distribution. You are 95% sure that a 95% confidence interval contains the true population value. For the same data, higher confidence requires a wider confidence interval.

confound the effects of two variables are said to be confounded if they are inseparable. This undesirable phenomenon is usually the result of poor study design.

continuous a variable is continuous if it can take any value in a particular range (i.e. it can take decimal values).

control group a group of subjects used in a study as a comparison with the group of primary interest.

correlation the correlation coefficient is a measure of the degree of linear association between two continuous variables. A value of +1 indicates perfect positive association, a value of −1 indicates perfect negative association, and a value of 0 indicates no linear association. The value is highly sensitive to a few abnormal data values.

cross-sectional study an observational study in which subjects are investigated at one point in time.

data numbers or values that are collected for analysis.

data dredging the highly undesirable practice of searching through data in an attempt to find an interesting result. It is sometimes called data fishing, and (to a lesser extent nowadays) data mining.

dependent variable a somewhat confusing term that is used in statistical modelling. When one variable is believed to influence another variable, the latter is called the dependent variable. It is sometimes called a response or outcome variable, and is plotted on the vertical axis of a graph.

dichotomous taking two possible values (i.e. binary).

discrete a variable is discrete if it can only take certain values. These are usually whole numbers (e.g. counts).

distribution distributions describe the histograms of whole populations. There are several distributions that are commonly used (e.g. the normal distribution).

double-blind a trial is double-blind if neither the subject nor the person conducting the assessment of the subject knows to which treatment group the subject has been allocated. Uses of the term vary.

EER experimental event rate – the rate at which an event occurs in the experimental group. It is a percentage.

equivalence study a study in which the objective is to show that two treatments are equivalent in outcome, as opposed to showing that one is superior to the other. The two types of study need to be designed differently.

estimate a value calculated from a sample when you are really interested in the value for the population. It is an informed guess!

experiment a comparative study in which the researchers are able to control the factor of interest. A typical example is a clinical trial in which one treatment is given to one group of subjects and another treatment is given to a second group of subjects. The researchers determine who receives which treatment.

factor a variable with (a few) discrete levels. The term is also used to describe a condition controlled by a researcher in an experiment (e.g. different treatments).

geometric mean a type of average, usually close to the median. It is related to the product of all of the data values. It occurs when positively skewed data have been transformed by taking logs before analysis.

histogram a chart that is used to represent continuous data. It consists of bars which are adjacent, and whose area is proportional to the frequency for that range of values.

independent two events are independent if knowing about one tells you nothing about the other.

intention-to-treat analysis in clinical trials subjects may drop out of the study or change treatment groups. An intention-to-treat analysis retains data from all such subjects in the group to which they were originally allocated. This is considered to be the correct way to deal with dropouts.

interaction an interaction exists between two variables or factors if the effect of one depends on the value of the other.

interquartile range the difference between the lower and upper quartiles, used to describe the variability in ordinal or skewed data.

interrupted time series a study in which subjects are studied over a period of time – before and then after an event or intervention of interest.

lie factor a number that is used to describe the fairness of graphs or charts. It is the ratio of the size of the apparent effect in the chart to the actual effect in the data. A lie factor of 1 denotes fairness.

Likert-type scale a scale on questionnaires where a subject is asked to what extent they agree with a statement.

linear association a linear association exists between two continuous variables if a reasonable amount of variability in one is explained by a straight-line equation with the other. The scatter plot will show points scattered around a straight line.

longitudinal study a study in which subjects are followed over time. Characteristics are measured at several points in time.

lower quartile the value below which 25% of the data lie.

lurking variable two variables may be highly correlated, but this does not mean that one directly influences the other. Sometimes there is a third (lurking) variable which influences each of them. Lurking variables are used to explain why strong correlations may not be evidence of causality.

mean an average value that is computed by adding together all of the values and dividing by the number of values. Colloquially it is called the average, although in statistics there are different types of average.

median the middle value in a set of data. It is used when describing skewed or ordinal data.

meta-analysis an analysis which combines the results from several studies (usually in a systematic review) to provide an overall analysis and confidence interval.

minimisation a non-random procedure (scorned by some researchers), sometimes used in RCTs to achieve balance of several groups with regard to a number of variables.

mode the most frequently occurring value, used to describe nominal or ordinal data.

model an equation relating two or more variables.

multiple testing the rather dangerous practice of performing several tests on the same set of data. This is particularly undesirable if the tests are thought of after the data have been collected.

mutually exclusive two events are mutually exclusive if they cannot both occur together.

negative prediction rate in diagnostic testing, the probability that you do not have the disease when the test is negative. The value of the negative prediction rate can be affected by the prevalence rate.

nominal a variable is nominal if it can take a set of values that are not ordered (e.g. ethnic origin).

non-parametric test a test which requires no distributional assumptions about the data.

normal distribution a symmetrical bell-shaped distribution that is often used to model data.

null hypothesis the hypothesis which states that there is no effect or difference. We assume that this hypothesis is true, and it is only rejected if there is a weight of evidence against it in the data.

observational study a non-experimental study in which subjects are observed. Examples include cohort and case–control studies.

odds ratio a ratio of odds in two groups, often used in case–control studies to estimate relative risk.

one-sided test a test in which the alternative hypothesis is that an effect or difference is in a particular direction (e.g. greater than zero). If you intend to use a one-sided test, you should say so at the design stage, and you must have very good reason to do so.

ordinal data in which the various values have a natural order.

outlier a value in a data set which appears to be a long way from the rest of the data. It may be an error or an unusual or interesting value.

parameter a value such as a population mean or standard deviation, which is seldom known. You usually take a sample from the population and estimate the value of such parameters. It is also the name for a constant in a model.

parametric test a statistical test which relies on the data having a particular distribution (often the normal distribution).

pie chart a circle that is divided into sections so that the area of each slice is proportional to the number represented. It is used when all subdivisions of the subject are being studied, and you want to show how the relative sizes of the subdivisions differ. Three-dimensional pie charts can be very misleading.

pilot study a small-scale study that is conducted in order to investigate the usefulness of some method or tool (e.g. a questionnaire) that you intend to use in the full-scale study.

placebo an inert substance, indistinguishable from the active drug, which is given to the control group. This enables both subjects and researchers to remain blinded to the treatment allocation.

population the entire set of subjects or items about which you want information.

positive prediction rate in diagnostic testing, the probability that you do have the disease when the test is positive. The value can be affected by the prevalence rate.

power the probability that you will find a statistically significant difference, using a statistical test, when that size of difference actually exists.

power calculation before starting a study you should estimate the size of the sample that you need in order to have high enough power to be able to detect a clinically significant effect. This process is called a power calculation.

predictor variable sometimes called an explanatory or (rather confusingly) independent variable. The variable that is plotted on the horizontal axis, and that is used in modelling to predict the values of the response variable.

probability a measure of how likely an event is. A value of $+1$ denotes certainty, and a value of 0 denotes impossibility.

prospective cohort study a study in which a group of subjects is followed forward in time. Usually the level of risk is measured first, and the subjects are monitored for development of a disease.

P-value very commonly misunderstood, this is the probability of observing a test statistic at least as extreme as that actually observed *if the null hypothesis is true*. A small P-value is interpreted as strong evidence against the null hypothesis. Confidence intervals are more informative than P-values.

random sample a sample chosen from the population by chance – each member has an equal chance of being selected.

randomisation the method of allocating subjects to treatments using the principle of chance.

randomised controlled trial (RCT) a study in which at least two treatment groups are studied, one of which is a control group. Randomisation is used to allocate the subjects to the treatment groups.

range the difference between the smallest and largest values in the data.

regression line a straight-line equation that is used to model the relationship between a response variable and one or more predictor variables.

relative risk the ratio of the risk of some event in one group relative to that in another group.

reliability a tool is said to be reliable if it consistently gives the same results.

repeated-measures study a study of subjects where more than one measure is taken on the same subject, usually over a period of time. Measures on the same subject will be correlated, so special methods of analysis are needed.

response variable sometimes called the outcome variable or the dependent variable. In plots it will be represented on the vertical axis. In modelling it is the variable being predicted by the model.

retrospective study an observational study in which subjects are chosen by disease status and then followed back in time in order to ascertain their exposure to a risk. Typically it is a case–control study.

RRR relative risk reduction – the percentage of the original risk that was eliminated by a treatment.

sample a set of people or items chosen for study from the population.

sampling frame the list of the entire population of interest, used to draw a sample.

scatter plot a graph showing the relationship between two continuous variables. Each symbol on the graph is determined by the pair of values of the variables.

sensitivity when using a diagnostic test, the percentage of people with the disease who will test positive.

significance level the probability of rejecting the null hypothesis when it is in fact true. A level of 5% is usually chosen.

single-blind a study in which the subjects are unaware of which treatment they are receiving. However, usage of the term is inconsistent. Some people use the term to refer to studies where the assessor, but not the subjects, are unaware of the treatment allocation.

skewness data are skewed if the histogram has a long tail on one side.

specificity when using a diagnostic test, the percentage of people without the disease who will test negative.

standard deviation a measure of spread or variability, used for continuous symmetrical data in conjunction with the mean.

standard error a measure of the uncertainty in an estimate from a sample.

statistic a value calculated from a sample (e.g. the sample mean).

stratified sampling a method of sampling that is used to compare subsets of a population. Samples are taken from each of the subsets rather than from the population as a whole.

survey an observational study that is used to find out the characteristics of a population. The method of sampling is critically important.

survival data data that arise from studies where the outcome of interest is the time until a particular event (often death). Censored data are often obtained from such a study.

systematic review a summary of all of the medical literature associated with a particular research question. The search for studies must be systematic and comprehensive.

test statistic a statistic that is calculated from a sample and used in a statistical test. An extreme value of a test statistic will result in a low P-value and thus rejection of the null hypothesis.

time-series plot a plot that shows the change in a variable or variables over time.

transformation if data are not normally distributed, they are sometimes transformed on to a different scale by a mathematical manipulation.

treatment group a group in a study that receives an active treatment which is under investigation.

two-sided test a test where the alternative hypothesis is that the effect of interest can be in either direction (e.g. where a drug can be worse or better than placebo).

type I error rejecting the null hypothesis when it is true (i.e. claiming to have found an effect that is not really there).

type II error failing to reject the null hypothesis when it is false (i.e. not finding an effect even though it is there).

upper quartile the value below which 75% of the data lie.

validation the process of checking whether a tool actually measures what it is supposed to measure.

variable a characteristic, subject to variability, that can be measured.

variance the value of the standard deviation squared. The standard deviation is much easier to understand.

VAS visual analogue scale – a line of fixed length (usually 10 cm) with extreme labels at the ends. Subjects are asked to place a mark such as a cross on the scale to correspond to their opinion or condition.

References

Preface

1   Wulff HR, Anderson B, Brandenhoff P and Guttler F (1987) What do doctors know about statistics? *Statist Med.* **6**: 3–10.

2   Berwick DM, Fineberg HV and Weinstein MC (1981) When doctors meet numbers. *Am J Med.* **71**: 991–8.

3   Altman DG and Bland JM (1991) Improving doctors' understanding of statistics. *J R Stat Soc.* **154**: 223–67.

4   Altman D (1991) *Practical Statistics for Medical Research.* Chapman and Hall, London.

5   Lindsay JK (1999) *Revealing Statistical Principles.* Edward Arnold, London.

6   Campbell M and Machin D (1993) *Medical Statistics. A Common-Sense Approach.* John Wiley & Sons, Chichester.

7   Bland M (1995) *An Introduction to Medical Statistics.* Oxford Medical Publications, Oxford.

8   Morris S (2000) *Statistics for the Terrified v4.0.* Radcliffe Medical Press, Oxford.

9   Nelder JA (1999) Statistics for the Millennium. From statistics to statistical science. *Statistician.* **48**: 257–69.

Chapter 1

1   Greenhalgh T (1997) How to read a paper: the Medline database. *BMJ.* **315**: 180–3.

2   Vickers AJ and de Craen AJ (2000) Why use placebos in clinical trials? A narrative review of the methodological literature. *J Clin Epidemiol.* **53**: 157–61.

3   Altman D (1991) *Practical Statistics for Medical Research.* Chapman and Hall, London.

4   Pocock SJ (1983) *Clinical Trials: a Practical Approach.* John Wiley & Sons, New York.

5   Senn S (1997) *Statistical Issues in Drug Development.* John Wiley & Sons, Chichester.

6   Senn SJ (1993) *Cross-Over Trials in Clinical Research.* John Wiley & Sons, Chichester.

7   Whitehead J (1997) *Design and Analysis of Sequential Clinical Trials.* John Wiley & Sons, Chichester.

8   Friedman LM, Furberg CD and DeMets DL (1996) *Fundamentals of Clinical Trials* (3e). Mosby Yearbook Publishers, St Louis, MO.

9   Clarke M and Oxman AD (eds) (2000) Cochrane Reviewers' Handbook 4.1 (updated June 2000). Section 6. In: *Review Manager (RevMan)* (computer program) *Version 4.1*. The Cochrane Collaboration, Oxford.

10 Khan HA and Sempos CT (1989) *An Introduction to Epidemiologic Methods.* Oxford University Press, Oxford.

11 Breslow NE and Day NE (1980) *Statistical Methods in Cancer Research. Volume I. The Analysis of Case–Control Studies.* International Agency for Research on Cancer, Lyon.

12 Breslow NE and Day NE (1987) *Statistical Methods in Cancer Research. Volume II. The Design and Analysis of Cohort Studies.* Oxford University Press/International Agency for Research on Cancer, Oxford.

13 Schlesselman JJ (1982) *Case–Control Studies. Design, Conduct, Analysis.* Oxford University Press, Oxford.

14 Moser CA and Kalton G (1972) *Survey Methods in Social Investigation* (2e). Basic Books, New York.

15 Sudman S (1976) *Applied Sampling.* Academic Press, London.

16 Barnett V (1991) *Sample Survey Principles and Methods.* Edward Arnold, London.

17 Lattimer V, George S, Thompson F *et al.* (1998) Safety and effectiveness of nurse telephone consultation in out-of-hours primary care: randomised controlled trial. *BMJ.* **317**: 1054–9.

18 Ong KLK, Ahmed ML, Emmett PM *et al.* (2000) Association between postnatal catch-up growth and obesity in childhood: prospective cohort study. *BMJ.* **320**: 967–71.

19 Tyssen R, Vaglum P, Grønvold NT and Ekeberg Ø (2000) The impact of job stress and working conditions on mental health problems among junior house-officers. A nationwide Norwegian prospective cohort study. *Med Educ.* **34**: 374–84.

20 Hawton K, Simkin S, Deeks JJ *et al.* (1999) Effects of a drug overdose in a television drama on presentations to hospital for self-poisoning: time series and questionnaire study. *BMJ.* **318**: 972–7.

21 Freedman DM, Dosemeci M and Alavanja MCR (2000) Mortality from multiple sclerosis and exposure to residential and occupational solar radiation: a case–control study based on death certificates. *Occup Env Med.* **57**: 418–21.

22 Jones JM, Lawson ML, Daneman D *et al.* (2000) Eating disorders in adolescent females with and without type I diabetes: cross-sectional study. *BMJ.* **320**: 1563–6.

23 Jones CM, O'Brien K, Blinkhorn AS and Rood RP (1997) Dentists' agreement on treatment of asymptomatic impacted third molar teeth: interview study. *BMJ.* **315**: 1204.

24   Bradbury A, Evans C, Allan P *et al.* (1999) What are the symptoms of varicose veins? Edinburgh vein study cross-sectional population survey. *BMJ.* **318**: 353–6.

Chapter 2

1   Tyssen R, Vaglum P, Grønvold NT and Ekeberg Ø (2000) The impact of job stress and working conditions on mental health problems among junior house-officers. A nationwide Norwegian prospective cohort study. *Med Educ.* **34**: 374–84.

2   Streiner DL and Norman GR (1995) *Health Measurement Scales. A Practical Guide to their Development and Use* (2e). Oxford University Press, Oxford.

3   McDowell I and Newell C (1987) *Measuring Health: A Guide to Rating Scales and Questionnaires.* Oxford University Press, Oxford.

4   Bowling A (1991) *Measuring Health: A Review of Quality of Life Measurement Scales.* Open University Press, Philadelphia, PA.

5   Bowling A (1995) *Measuring Disease.* Open University Press, Buckingham.

6   Wilkin D, Hallam L and Doggett MA (1992) *Measures of Need and Outcome for Primary Health Care.* Oxford University Press, Oxford.

Chapter 3

1   Tufte ER (1983) *The Visual Display of Quantitative Information.* Graphics Press, Cheshire, CT.

2   Huff D (1954) *How to Lie with Statistics.* WW Norton & Company, New York.

3   Elting L, Martin CG, Cantor SB and Rubenstein EB (1999) Influence of data display on physician investigators' decision to stop trials: prospective trial with repeated measures. *BMJ.* **318**: 1527–31.

4   Wyatt JC (1999) Same information, different decisions: format counts. *BMJ.* **318**: 1501–2.

Chapter 4

1   Hawton K, Simkin S, Deeks JJ *et al.* (1999) Effects of a drug overdose in a television drama on presentations to hospital for self-poisoning: time series and questionnaire study. *BMJ.* **318**: 972–7.

2   Lattimer V, George S, Thompson F *et al.* (1998) Safety and effectiveness of nurse telephone consultation in out-of-hours primary care: randomised controlled trial. *BMJ.* **317**: 1054–9.

3   Jones JM, Lawson ML, Daneman D *et al.* (2000) Eating disorders in adolescent females with and without type I diabetes: cross-sectional study. *BMJ.* **320**: 1563–6.

4   Thompson SG and Barber JA (2000) How should cost data in pragmatic randomised trials be analysed? *BMJ.* **320**: 1197–200.

5   Altman D (1991) *Practical Statistics for Medical Research.* Chapman and Hall, London.

6   Bland M (1987) *An Introduction to Medical Statistics.* Oxford University Press, Oxford.

7   Hollis S and Campbell F (1999) What is meant by intention-to-treat analysis? Survey of published randomised controlled trials. *BMJ.* **319**: 670–4.

Chapter 5

1   Ong KLK, Ahmed ML, Emmett PM *et al.* (2000) Association between postnatal catch-up growth and obesity in childhood: prospective cohort study. *BMJ.* **320**: 967–71.

Chapter 6

1   Lattimer V, George S, Thompson F *et al.* (1998) Safety and effectiveness of nurse telephone consultation in out-of-hours primary care: randomised controlled trial. *BMJ.* **317**: 1054–9.

2   Hawton K, Simkin S, Deeks JJ *et al.* (1999) Effects of a drug overdose in a television drama on presentations to hospital for self-poisoning: time series and questionnaire study. *BMJ.* **318**: 972–7.

3   Gardner MJ and Altman DG (eds) (1989) *Statistics with Confidence.* BMJ Publications, London.

4   Altman DG (1985) Comparability of randomised groups. *Statistician.* **34**: 125–36.

5   Altman DG and Bland JM (1995) Statistics notes – absence of evidence is not evidence of absence. *BMJ.* **311**: 485.

6   Senn S (1997) *Statistical Issues in Drug Development.* John Wiley & Sons, Chichester.

Chapter 7

1   Ong KLK, Ahmed ML, Emmett PM *et al.* (2000) Association between postnatal catch-up growth and obesity in childhood: prospective cohort study. *BMJ.* **320**: 967–71.

2   Streiner DL and Norman GR (1995) *Health Measurement Scales. A Practical Guide to Their Development and Use* (2e). Oxford University Press, Oxford.

3   Dunn G (1989) *Design and Analysis of Reliability Studies. The Statistical Evaluation of Measurement Errors.* Edward Arnold, London.

4   Nguyen M, Revel M and Dougados M (1997) Prolonged effects of 3-week therapy in a spa resort on lumbar spine, knee and hip osteoarthritis: follow-up after 6 months. A randomized controlled trial. *Br J Rheumatol.* **36**: 77–81.

Chapter 8

1   Anderson B (1990) *Methodological Errors in Medical Research: an Incomplete Catalogue.* Blackwell Scientific Publications, Oxford.

2   Altman D and Bland JM (1991) Improving doctors' understanding of statistics. *J R Stat Soc.* **154**: 223–67.

3   White AR and Ernst E (1999) A systematic review of randomized controlled trials of acupuncture for neck pain. *Rheumatology.* **38**: 143–7.

4   Atkins D, Crawford F, Edwards J and Lambert M (1999) A systematic review of treatments for the painful heel. *Rheumatology.* **38**: 968–73.

5   Butcher HC and Schmidt JG (1993) Does ultrasound scanning improve outcome in pregnancy? Meta-analysis of various outcome measures. *BMJ.* **307**: 13–17.

6   Woodward M (1999) *Epidemiology: Study Design and Data Analysis.* Chapman and Hall, London.

7   Greenhalgh T (1997) How to read a paper: the Medline database. *BMJ.* **315**: 180–3.

8   Sackett DL, Straus SE, Richardson WS, Rosenberg W and Haynes RB (2000) *Evidence-Based Medicine. How to Practise and Teach EBM* (2e). Churchill Livingstone, London (http://hiru.mcmaster.ca/ebm.htm)

9   Altman DG (1996) Better reporting of randomised controlled trials: the CONSORT statement. *BMJ.* **313**: 570–1.

10 Greenhalgh T (1997) *How to Read a Paper: the Basics of Evidence-Based Medicine.* BMJ Publishing Group, London.

11 Altman D (1991) *Practical Statistics for Medical Research.* Chapman and Hall, London.

12 Gore SM and Altman DG (eds) (1982) *Statistics in Practice.* British Medical Association, London.

13 Elwood M (1998) *Critical Appraisal of Epidemiological Studies and Clinical Trials.* Oxford Medical Publications, Oxford.

14 Chambers R and Booth E (2001) *Clinical Effectiveness and Clinical Governance Made Easy* (2e). Radcliffe Medical Press, Oxford.

15   Lattimer V, George S, Thompson F *et al.* (1998) Safety and effectiveness of nurse telephone consultation in out-of-hours primary care: randomised controlled trial. *BMJ.* **317**: 1054–9.

16   Ong KLK, Ahmed ML, Emmett PM *et al.* (2000) Association between postnatal catch-up growth and obesity in childhood: prospective cohort study. *BMJ.* **320**: 967–71.

17   Tyssen R, Vaglum P, Grønvold NT and Ekeberg Ø (2000) The impact of job stress and working conditions on mental health problems among junior house-officers. A nationwide Norwegian prospective cohort study. *Med Educ.* **34**: 374–84.

18   Hawton K, Simkin S, Deeks JJ *et al.* (1999) Effects of a drug overdose in a television drama on presentations to hospital for self-poisoning: time series and questionnaire study. *BMJ.* **318**: 972–7.

19   Freedman DM, Dosemeci M and Alavanja MCR (2000) Mortality from multiple sclerosis and exposure to residential and occupational solar radiation: a case–control study based on death certificates. *Occup Environ Med.* **57**: 418–21.

Glossary

1   Sackett DL, Straus SE, Richardson WS, Rosenberg W and Haynes RB (2000) *Evidence-Based Medicine. How to Practise and Teach EBM* (2e). Churchill Livingstone, London.

2   Pereira-Maxwell F (1998) *A–Z of Medical Statistics: a Companion for Critical Appraisal.* Edward Arnold, London.

3   Everitt B (1995) *Dictionary of Statistics in the Medical Sciences.* Cambridge University Press, Cambridge.

Index